The Nature of Prejudice

This book offers a critical synthesis of social psychology's contribution to the study of contemporary racism, and proposes a critical reframing of our understanding of prejudice in European society today. Chapters place a special emphasis on the diversity and intensity of prejudices against Romani people in a liberal, progressive, decent, enlarged Europe. Chapters ask how we can reconcile the European creed of law, justice and freedom for all, with social and political practices that exclude and degrade Romani people.

This volume addresses the need for a deeper recognition of societal foundations of ideologies of moral exclusion, and calls for a closer and thorough investigation of prejudices that stem from the societal transformation, diminution or denial of moral worth of human beings (and the various conditions and contexts that create and promote it). By opening new intellectual dialogues, the book reinvigorates a renewed social psychology of racism, and creates a broader foundation for the exploration of active paradoxes at the heart of the social expression of prejudice in liberal democracies.

The Nature of Prejudice is essential reading for academics, researchers and postgraduate students interested in both the quantitative and qualitative study of discrimination, inequality and social exclusion.

Cristian Tileagă is Senior Lecturer in Social Psychology and member of the Discourse and Rhetoric Group at Loughborough University, UK.

Explorations in Social Psychology series
Books in this series:

Rhetoric, Ideology and Social Psychology
Essays in honour of Michael Billig
Edited by Charles Antaki and Susan Condor

Terrorism, Trauma and Psychology
A multilevel victim perspective of the Bali bombings
Gwendoline Patricia Brookes, Julie Ann Pooley and Jaya Earnest

Psychological War Trauma and Society
Like a hidden wound
Irit Keynan

The Nature of Prejudice
Society, discrimination and moral exclusion
Cristian Tileagă

Discursive Psychology
Classic and contemporary issues
Edited by Cristian Tileagă and Elizabeth Stokoe

The Nature of Prejudice

Society, discrimination and moral exclusion

Cristian Tileagă

Routledge
Taylor & Francis Group
LONDON AND NEW YORK

First published 2016
by Routledge
27 Church Road, Hove, East Sussex, BN3 2FA

and by Routledge
711 Third Avenue, New York, NY 10017

Routledge is an imprint of the Taylor & Francis Group, an informa business

British Library Cataloguing in Publication data
A catalogue record for this book is available from the British Library

Library of Congress Cataloguing in Publication data
Tileagă, Cristian, 1975–
The nature of prejudice : society, discrimination and moral exclusion / Cristian Tileagă.
pages cm
1. Marginality, Social–European Union countries. 2. Racism–European Union countries. 3. Social psychology–European Union countries. 4. Romanies–Social conditions–European Union countries. I. Title.
HN380.Z9M2683 2016
305.800947–dc23
2014048884

ISBN: 978-0-415-83985-3 (hbk)
ISBN: 978-0-203-77069-6 (ebk)

Typeset in Galliard
by Out of House Publishing

MIX
Paper from responsible sources
FSC® C013056
FSC www.fsc.org

Printed and bound in Great Britain by
TJ International Ltd, Padstow, Cornwall

To Eva Tileagă, my grandmother, who taught me how to challenge my own prejudices

Contents

Preface and acknowledgements

How to pursue the European project and respond to the challenges of globalization without excluding people? How to treat others who are alike (European citizens) but also, essentially, unlike 'us'? These are some of the moral quandaries that European governments are trying to address, in the name of a professed European creed of law, justice and freedom for all.

Yet, in an enlarged Europe, the European creed of law, justice and freedom for all does not seem to be extended to all. The current European project of accommodating diversity without troubling national sovereignty does not seem to find an appropriate place for Romani people's worth and aspirations. The current European project of accommodating diversity shows how fragile human dignity is. This is a book about the diversity and intensity of prejudices against Romani people in a liberal, progressive, decent, Europe. This is a book about what might be described as the last acceptable form of racism in European societies – racism against Romani people.

Contemporary European prejudices against Romani people, ranging from the subtle to the extreme, show that democratic and liberal values of decency, tolerance, reasonableness, are sometimes not enough to erode (a history of) intolerance. When explaining, or trying to respond to, the challenges that racism poses in European liberal democracies, we tend to be swayed by either manifestations of unadulterated hostility or unconditional sympathy, whilst, sometimes, forgetting to consider the views and experiences of the decent (tolerant, reasonable) 'middle'. We are more inclined to believe that the prejudices of the decent 'middle' are the outcome of implicit, automatic, unconscious bias. Yet, when one turns to the predicament of Romani people in Europe one observes that the presence of Romanies creates marked moral uneasiness for the vast majority of people who see themselves belonging to the decent 'middle'. European societies are engaged in a dialogue about the moral status that should be assigned to Romani people. The decent 'middle' (which covers both lay and elite views and experiences with difference) sustains this dialogue about the moral status of Romanies.

In this book I propose a critical reframing of understanding prejudice and racism in society: a shift from prejudice as antipathy to prejudice as harm inflicted by indignity. I argue that one cannot appreciate fully the societal, collective conversation about the moral status of Romanies in European societies if one does not explore closely the nature of prejudices that stem from the diminution or denial of people's moral worth and the societal conditions and contexts that perpetuate them. Social psychology needs to renew its intellectual dialogue with kindred social science fields to create broader foundations for the exploration of the various, active paradoxes lodged at the heart of the social expression of prejudice in liberal democracies, and the genesis and cultural, societal anchoring of prejudices that devalue people.

The seeds of this book were planted between 2001 and 2004 whilst conducting doctoral research at Loughborough University on majority group prejudices against Romanies. I owe a special debt of gratitude to Michael Billig (my supervisor at the time, and now colleague in the Department of Social Sciences), Susan Condor, Charles Antaki, Jovan Byford, Geraldo Gomes, Sabina Mihelj, and to current and past members of the Discourse and Rhetoric Group at Loughborough. This project began with papers written for *Discourse & Society*, *British Journal of Social Psychology*, *Journal of Community and Applied Social Psychology* and *Ethnicities*. More recently, I have continued to explore some of the issues developed in this book in another monograph *Political Psychology: Critical Perspectives* (published by Cambridge University Press), and in a chapter written for *Rhetoric, Ideology and Social Psychology: Essays in Honour of Michael Billig* (edited by Charles Antaki and Susan Condor, and published by Routledge). I am grateful to John Wiley and Sons, Sage Publications, Cambridge University Press and Routledge, for permitting me to reuse and rewrite material in the present form. Here, I attempt to integrate the various threads from my previous work by looking for a more adequate, encompassing, social scientific framework for exploring anti-Romani prejudices and racism.

Prompted by the desire to keep this book accessible and readable I had to be selective in my choice of focus. It is impossible to do justice to such a vast and complex subject (the nature of the Romani predicament in Europe) within the confines of a conventional academic monograph. This book does not contain statistics on key social indicators of social exclusion nor does it have a separate chapter on the well-documented history of Romani persecution in Europe. There is a wealth of data publicly available elsewhere, and a plethora of excellent works on Romani history, some of which I have used here. The book is addressed to academics and researchers interested in both the quantitative and qualitative study of discrimination, inequality and social exclusion; students undertaking masters or doctoral studies in social psychology, political psychology, political science, peace studies, media and communication, sociology or cognate disciplines; think tanks and non-profit NGOs active in the fight against racism in Europe; Roma organizations; and journalists, politicians, advocates and researchers of key policy domains including education, housing, healthcare, immigration and crime.

I hope that this project will elicit further, and perhaps deeper, consideration of some of the issues highlighted here. Because I am a social psychologist I gave priority to a central social psychological theme – the idea that problems of prejudice and hostility in society are irreducible to flawed reasoning, irrational propensities and/or attitudinal negativity. In writing this book I returned to one of the classics of the field – Gordon W. Allport's *The Nature of Prejudice* (1954). The title, but also, more importantly, the spirit of this book is indebted to that wonderful tome, which contains some of the most productive paradoxes of social psychology. Although Allport is rightly seen as the father of cognitive studies of prejudice, he was also very much aware that it is society and cultural assumptions that can alter or transform our own ideas about other people's moral worth, our evaluations of their vulnerability and our judgements about society's role in oppression.

This is a book that proposes as an alternative a critical, cultural analysis of societal presuppositions and mechanisms of enacting moral exclusion by transforming or altering people's worth and dignity. The transformation, diminution or denial of Romani people's moral worth is a product of discursive, symbolic, material, legal, political tropes of modern/liberal democratic societies. Romanies are not only actively degraded by the societies in which they dwell; they are also constantly reminded of their modified worth and degraded status.

Introduction

Prejudice as an interpretive concept

Prejudice is an interpretive concept. People disagree about what prejudice is. They disagree about its sources, the forms it takes, its intensities and social impact. Social psychologists, as well as lay members of society, are at pains to locate the concept (and its manifestations) in some set of distinct descriptions that, purportedly, best capture its nature. Social psychological theory underpins or feeds into the substance of these descriptions.

This book explores the contribution of social psychological theory to understanding prejudice as an interpretive concept. This is a book about the conversations that every society conducts with itself regarding the fate of those designated as Others. This book focuses on the specific conversation that (Western and Eastern) European societies are now conducting: a conversation about the *place* and *fate* of the Roma minority in Europe. I will be arguing that this is a conversation not only about how societies organize and protect themselves against aliens, immigrants, etc., but also a conversation about human worth, dignity, compassion and dilemmas at the heart of liberal democracies. Various commentators and national and European politicians are warning that European societies are now facing perhaps one of the most tragic dilemmas of our times: How to protect citizens from the undesirable effects of globalization (Barroso, 2014)?

In the case of the Roma minority in Europe, we are witnessing, with extraordinary frequency, how a desire to uphold the values of sympathy coexists with a desire to control the flux of people, erect barriers and enforce boundaries; how toughness and conservatism coexist with reasonableness and humanitarianism. Following Fassin (2005), I will be arguing that liberal democracies are mechanisms of domination as well as empowerment. There is a foundational tension at the heart of liberal democracies: a tension between domination and empowerment, exclusion and sympathy, which regulates the perpetuation and expression of tolerance and intolerance, as two faces of the same coin.

For social psychologists, prejudice is both a natural and universal fact of life reflecting our inner psychology as well as exceptional, particularistic, unique. The automaticity of stereotypes or the natural distinction or neat categorization between in-groups and out-groups in minimal group settings are examples of the former, whilst the case of extreme prejudice and genocide are examples of the latter. However, social psychologists have been less concerned with constructing a cultural critique of prejudice as a socio-cultural phenomenon, socio-communicative and experiential product with origins in the cultural, political and legal organization of societies. Part of constructing a cultural critique of prejudice entails the recognition of what research, experience and history show – that not all prejudices are the same: they are culturally and ideologically situated, their expression depends on a complex interplay of socio-cultural, political and ideological factors.

Although, since Allport's seminal work on prejudice (Allport, 1954), social psychologists have shown that a psychological exploration of the individual mind needs to be linked to societal and socio-cultural levels of analysis (e.g. Jost and Hamilton, 2005), they are, arguably, less interested in researching the tensions, contradictions, ambiguities of democratic regimes and governance that foster forms of domination (intolerance) as well as sympathy (tolerance). They pay less attention to the cultural nature of the 'stock' of everyday and elite beliefs about morality, transgression and justice, that every society bequeaths its members (Opotow, 2007).

Intolerance and tolerance as societal tropes

What we broadly call 'tolerance' and 'intolerance' is a social product of liberal democracies. This book is an invitation to identify the means by which we can treat, research and respond to prejudice as social and cultural product. This makes sense for at least one fundamental reason – we experience, witness or judge prejudice as a pervasive cultural dimension. The tropes of intolerance and tolerance are cultural/societal tropes. Our desire to fight prejudice head on, or, in some cases, our ambivalence towards prejudice, is a cultural product of the societies in which we dwell.

In the social psychology of prejudice, the term 'society' does not seem to resonate as deeply as notions of 'group', 'groups', 'intergroup relations'. As Bar-Tal and Teichman (2005) argue, 'the term [society] has almost disappeared from the vocabulary of mainstream social psychology' (p. 8). Social psychologists do not feel the need to provide their readers with a working definition of what social scientists call 'society', and are 'preoccupied mostly with specific, microlevel research questions and refrains from looking at real-life issues in a holistic way' (ibid., p. 2). 'Society' is, sometimes, simply the background against which research is conducted, without direct consequences for the way findings are interpreted. Researching prejudice *in* society entails researching macro-contexts holistically, and approaching conventional individual phenomena as societal phenomena, including, but not limited to, 'agents of socialization, societal channels of communication, social institutions, and cultural products' (ibid., p. 8).

I argue that, in order to understand prejudice as a natural reflection of our inner psychology and its exceptionality or context-bound uniqueness, social psychology needs to incorporate a reflexive metatheory of 'society' in its theorizing and empirical approaches. This reflexive metatheory would treat 'society' not only as a meaningful entity of belonging and identification, but, more importantly, as a reflexive product of meaning-making in spaces and places where different orders – discursive, material, civic, legal, ethnic, economic and political – intersect and feed into each other. For this reflexive metatheory of 'society' social psychologists may need to turn to the social sciences, especially to currents and strands of scholarship in sociology, social theory and anthropology (Boltanski, 2011, 2012; Fassin, 2005, 2008; Wacquant, 2008). As Margaret Wetherell has argued recently, social psychologists are perhaps more attuned to making inter- or cross-disciplinary connections and 'more used to treading the shaky bridge between conventional psychology and the social sciences' (2012, p. 11).

Here, I contend that a renewed impetus in the social psychology of prejudice and racism can exploit meaningfully the 'societal' gaps and absences in mainstream social psychology. A social psychology of prejudice and racism needs a stronger intellectual commitment to researching and fighting prejudice as a cultural product of liberal democratic societies. This may lead to a better appreciation of the idea that researching prejudice and racism should not be limited to conceiving it as a fundamentally psychological problem. There is a need to relocate prejudice from people's mindsets into the midst of active societal/collective thinking. Social psychologists should be able to describe this activity of collective thinking without unique recourse to individual psychology (Tileagă, 2014). They need to work towards fulfilling the promise of a much older project in social psychology (and the social sciences): reconciling the thinking individual with the socio-cultural context in which they are operating. This is not exclusively a (social) psychological project, but also, resolutely, historical, sociological and anthropological too.

Experiences with such a project can be more easily found in other disciplines such as sociology, social theory, anthropology or history. Social psychology, however, is not without its attempts at integration. Gordon W. Allport's *The Nature of Prejudice* is, perhaps, the most notable. Allport has given us the single most thorough and persuasive account of prejudice as an interpretive concept. He is seen by contemporary social psychologists as a direct influence for a variety of topics and issues in the social psychology of prejudice (Dovidio *et al.*, 2005). Although his book is written in a pronounced psychological vein, Allport was very much aware of the risks involved in not taking into account historical and societal contexts. According to Allport, 'prejudice *is* something and *does* something. It is not the invention of liberals. Its importance in society merely adds urgency to what is in any case a basic psychological problem' (1950, p. 6, emphasis in original). Although Allport considered prejudice to be a problem of the individual, he contended that it is also a problem conterminous to 'social living'. Allport's contention echoes a sociological and anthropological perspective on prejudice (and racism in general) where prejudices are part and parcel of 'common and socialized experience' (Memmi, 2000, p. 30), and their source is 'lived experience itself' (ibid., p. 22).

Although Allport considered that 'ethnic prejudice is an antipathy based upon a faulty and inflexible generalization' (1954, p. 9), he also viewed the issue of prejudice as one of 'multiple causation'. Understanding the dynamic of prejudice entailed the understanding of inner and outer forces that reach 'behind and beyond the individual' (Allport, 1950, p. 17). Allport's emphasis on multiple causation echoes, again, anthropological descriptions of racism as social and cultural force: 'racism ... *attacks along many fronts and in many forms*, deploying whatever is at hand, and even what is not, inventing when the need arises' (Memmi, 2000, p. 78, emphasis in original).

Allport also recognized that prejudices, although psychological in origin, have a history. Without understanding the history of societies, their social and political organization, their intrinsic contradictions, both subtle and blatant forms of prejudice would be 'almost unintelligible' (Allport, 1950, p. 21). When Allport wrote his *Nature of Prejudice*, he wrote it not only as a social psychologist with an interest in prejudice, but perhaps also as an American citizen pained by his own country's burden of historical prejudice. He believed that the various insights of psychological science could contribute to solving national and universal dilemmas and burdens of historical prejudice. He has been proved mostly right by his exegesis, but, arguably, more effort needs to be spent on exploring the productive paradoxes and gaps in his work.

When one considers the continuous, historical prejudice and discrimination against Romani people in Europe (see Fraser, 1992 for an excellent account), it does not take much to notice its complex societal anchoring and the variety of ideological consequences stemming from that. As Allport himself suggested, one cannot understand the basic psychological problem of prejudice without taking into account a society's social, political and legal organization and functioning, its anthropological model of the person, and its history, traditions and symbolism of prejudice. Yet, one can identify a foundational paradox in Allport's work. Allport recognized the complexity of prejudices, although he continued to believe in the power of individual psychology and the universalist promise of psychology. He knew too well that to reduce prejudices to a set of psychological explanations would mean to miss the complexity of prejudices in (liberal) democracies. He only partially embraced the idea that any socio-psychological analysis of prejudice should include a historical and anthropological evaluation of a society's (or societies') creed and its (discriminatory and exclusionary) practices. Theorizing prejudice as 'a basic psychological problem' no longer seems to provide a satisfactory and comprehensive intellectual *appui* needed for researching the complex *nature* of specific contemporary prejudices.

As Jews before them, the Roma and their presence raises questions and puzzles that cannot be approached satisfactorily within existing social scientific frameworks. With extraordinary regularity, elite and lay discourse presents the Roma as a 'problem' without a 'solution'. Being cast as a 'problem' that calls for a solution, the Roma are not regarded any more as moral subjects, on the same moral footing as other members of society. Although, as Stewart argues, 'the plight of the Roma is truly Europe's plight' (2012b, p. 23), disquieting evidence shows that Europe still fails to protect the Roma from racist violence (Amnesty International, 2014). The plight of the Roma is perhaps the most visible symptom of what French philosopher Alain Finkielkraut (2013) called 'le défi contemporain du vivre-ensemble' (the contemporary challenge of living-together), part of a more general European malaise generally known as the 'crisis of integration'. As Yaron Matras argues:

> the Roms present us with a paradigmatic dilemma. They have no fixed territory but are dispersed ... Rather than having a territorial base or allegiance towards the symbols and institutions of a particular state, what defines Romani identity is a distinct language, a set of values and beliefs, a form of family organization and a particular outlook on the relations between their own community and the outside world.
>
> (2014, p. 22)

One of my goals in writing this book was to try to offer an account of how social psychology might engage with the paradigmatic dilemma identified by Matras, by opening a dialogue with other fields such as sociology and anthropology. In conversation with other scholarly fields, social psychology can offer a more confident, wide-ranging and critical approach to debates around the nature of societal prejudices in general, and anti-Roma prejudices in particular.

Prejudice as indignity

Understanding the nature of societal prejudices presents theoretical and empirical problems. How can we engage with prejudices that can be understood/perceived simultaneously as individual/personal, social, discursive and historical? What might be the best way forward? I would like to suggest that the problem lies with our current definitions of prejudice and discrimination and the (operational) nature of these definitions. The working definition of prejudice that most social psychologists use is an operational definition, a definition that says more about how real-life manifestations of prejudice *fit* existing psychological models or are described by a range of psychological variables or mental predispositions, rather than what is the *social meaning* of prejudice. Yet, prejudice is both an individual and collective phenomenon; it is neither expressed nor experienced in a social vacuum. I return to Allport to show how a definition of prejudice and discrimination around notions of dignity and worth in social relations may support a deeper understanding of the quandary of contemporary prejudices. The simplest and the most powerful definition of discrimination is offered by Allport (1954) – any behaviour that denies 'individuals or groups equality of treatment which they may wish' (p. 50). This is a definition that alludes to a dimension of aspirational worth, and dignity in social relations. According to Allport, discrimination is the resulting inequality based on differences of esteem (and respect). Interestingly, his definition seems more like a sociological, modern definition of discrimination, rather than a psychological one. Discrimination is wrong because it stifles public recognition of someone's social *worth*. Allport's definition also points to a fundamental human motivation of striving for equality of worth, respect, esteem.

One could draw parallels between Allport's definition and sociologists' concerns with 'status'. I am less concerned here with the notion of 'status' as used and defined by sociologists.[1] Although the notion of 'status' refers to 'inequality based on differences in honor, esteem, and respect' and can help us understand 'how much people care about their sense of being *valued* by others and the society to which they belong' (Ridgeway, 2014, p. 2, emphasis in original), it is used to understand more normative rather than ethical aspects of how vertical and horizontal social relations work. To understand the subtle mechanisms by which inequality is created and reproduced in society, I argue that one needs to move, paradoxically, beyond inequality as a status-driven normative framework. This is especially the case if one wishes to understand some of the foundational ethical quandaries and moral paradoxes of advanced/liberal democracies that arise from the tension between a society's creed and its practices.

Whether we are looking at gender, race or ethnicity, direct or subtle refusal of equality of treatment can have pernicious consequences leading to indignity. This does not mean that the meaning of in/dignity is the same in each case. As Habermas argues, the importance of human dignity 'extends beyond the vertical relation between individual citizens and the state and permeates the horizontal relations among individuals and groups' (2012, p. 80).

Legal and moral philosophers contend that 'acts are wrong if they insult the dignity of others' (Dworkin, 2013, p. 204). In its widest acceptation, dignity can be conceived as a 'value which is held universally and applies to all human beings' inherent and intrinsic worth' (Misztal, 2012, p. 101). According to Habermas, the notion of human dignity is not 'an empty placeholder ... that lumps a multiplicity of different phenomena together, but the moral "source" from which all of the basic rights derive their substance' (2012, p. 75). He also argues that 'the idea of human dignity is the conceptual hinge which connects the morality of equal respect for everyone with positive law and democratic lawmaking' (ibid., p. 81). When we talk about dignity and social justice in the same sentence, we also bring into view people's rights to self-determination and self-definition, and, more generally, people's rights (and desire) to be treated fairly and equitably by others and in the face of the law.

Human dignity does not operate solely as universalistic value principle. Human dignity is also a conceptual hinge for more particularistic constituents of morality that are upshots of everyday social practices. The democratic ideal represented by the nation-state is that of the organic community and participatory citizenship. Anything that disrupts it is cast aside. Under the framework of community and citizenship, human dignity turns, sometimes, into one of the most vulnerable aspects of democratic practice. Nation-states protect the human dignity of their 'citizens' through legal, political and economic mechanisms that, in certain conditions, refuse dignity to others. Nation-states create 'tests of worth' for aliens, refugees, strangers, whose 'format' they are, unfortunately, not able to change (see Boltanski and Thévenot, 2006 [1991]).

To understand prejudice as indignity implies tying the study of prejudice (and of its nature) to a constellation of conceptions and hypotheses accreting to the notion of *worth*. It perhaps makes sense to research prejudice as harm inflicted by indignity when one notices that exclusionary practices directed at those designated as Others (immigrants, asylum seekers, Roma, etc.) are all instances where people's social *worth* is modified, altered, transformed, and where harm is the *product* of modifying, altering, transforming people's social worth.

The historical and contemporary case of elite and everyday discourse directed at the Roma minority in Western and Eastern Europe is a conspicuous example of prejudice inflicted by indignity. The various calls for and cases of sterilization of the Roma in some European countries, their forced removal or relocation from town centres and private or public spaces, or declarations by public figures that Roma are 'not fit to live among people', or that they 'are animals and behave like animals', are only a few examples of deliberate attempts at altering, transforming the worth of the Roma minority, refusing them the dignity that other people take for granted, and thus removing them from the domain of moral acceptability. The current European project of accommodating diversity without troubling national sovereignty does not seem to find an appropriate place for Roma's (European) aspirations.

It is tempting to relegate these positions to the 'extreme' or to what Taguieff has called 'barbarism', as even 'those destined to barbarism are also products of modern democratic society' (1987, p. 154). The idea of prejudice as indignity is not just about the forms and consequences of extreme forms of social hostility. It is also about understanding the social and political ramifications of refusal/denial of dignity as a product of modern/liberal democratic society, and the various conditions and contexts that create and promote it. To the great majority of Europeans, the presence of the Roma creates marked moral uneasiness, and generates a variety of reactions, debates and calls for action.

National parliaments, European institutions and local councillors' meetings are in thrall to an unfolding argument about the moral status that should be assigned to the Roma. The European Union and member states are looking for a 'European solution' to the 'problems' of the Roma. The increased presence and visibility of the Roma in Europe has shaken Europe's self-fashioned cosmopolitan image of tolerance and inclusion. The Roma are the new face of marginality and poverty that triggers many moral-political dilemmas, stirs passions and unsettles the conventional management of social problems. The Roma embody a marginality that, as Wacquant argues, stands 'ahead of us ... etched on the horizon of the becoming of contemporary societies' (2008, p. 232).

Majorities allocate themselves the right 'to the ethical culture they deem best' (Dworkin, 2013, p. 370). Anyone that does not seem to tally with the accepted 'ethical culture' is ostracized, insulted, shunned, shown to be 'deficient' in the motivational and aspirational schemes of society. The line separating dignity from indignity is extremely precarious, especially when one is classed as 'different' or when one is described as an 'alien', 'foreigner', 'asylum seeker', or simply when one is a national of a country with the 'wrong' credentials or reputation. Although nation-states have a 'sovereign responsibility to treat each person in their power with equal concern and respect' (ibid., p. 321), the active 'definition' of different categories of persons and collectives possessing particular/definite characteristics invests them with different worth. At the same time, nation-states also reserve the right to enact policies that, in some cases, constitute a direct denial of equal concern and respect, and of the democratic principles on which the democratic structures and politics of modern democratic states and unions are based (e.g. freedom of movement). Indignity is not only social but also 'territorial' (Wacquant, 2008). There is a social but also a 'spatial patterning of inequality'. Separation, isolation, confinement '*radicalizes* the objective and subjective reality of ... exclusion' (ibid., p. 198, emphasis in original). Territorial indignity adds to a long list of 'stamps of dishonour' (ibid.) that make suffering visible, and enhance acute feelings of indignity.

A framework for critical analysis

An 'intricate web of labels and attitudes' meets anyone who wishes to understand the Roma (Matras, 2014). Social psychological analyses of prejudice and racism have largely ignored the Roma. Each chapter in this book is concerned with the limitations, as well as the promises, of social psychological approaches in addressing the quandary of anti-Roma prejudices. I will be arguing that, although social psychology has made extraordinary inroads, it is still quite limited in its explanatory reach of societal phenomena and social problems that, ostensibly, do not seem to fit some of its current disciplinary models. I draw on a variety of data sources (semi-structured interviews with majority group members, newspaper reports, news interviews and TV debates, Internet forums and social media, as well as settings where Roma themselves construct and manage their own representations of their ethnic identity) to argue for the need of a deeper recognition of the societal foundations of moral exclusionary ideologies in real-world contexts.

My aim is to outline the basis for an account of what I call 'critical analysis'. This is an approach that tries to understand the social reality and consequences of prejudice, racism and discrimination, through a framework steeped in a more general and richer metatheory of society than that offered by contemporary social psychological approaches. Critical analysis is not a version of established approaches to the study of racism like critical discourse analysis (van Dijk, 1993) or societal psychology (Howarth, 2004). By 'critical' I mean the potential of working with and within frameworks that conceive prejudice, racism and discrimination as a social and cultural system, firmly lodged in (and influenced by) the historic and current democratic social, political, legal order. Analysis is 'critical' insofar as it addresses societal dilemmas, tensions and contradictions that are 'ordinarily invisible' (Opotow, 2011), yet influence how liberal democracies organize themselves and construct their own collective social mechanisms for including and excluding people.

I identify three theoretical-conceptual hermeneutic principles that make up the core of critical analysis. The claims sketched here are developed in Chapter 1, and across the book as a whole.

The first principle is based on the recognition that prejudice, racism and discrimination are inherent social and cultural creations, aspects of collective life. They are achieved through words, images, symbols and social and material practices. Social and moral inclusion and exclusion reflect societal dynamics and are sourced in the complex social imaginary of societies (the socially shared 'stock' of prejudices, stereotypes, lay assumptions about group and ethnic categories, morality and transgression) and the ways in which individuals, groups and communities act on themselves and others, thus recognizing, or modifying, altering, transforming, each other's moral worth (Boltanski and Thévenot, 2006 [1991]).

The second, related, principle concerns the location of the answers to the moral, practical and political quandaries posed by the variety, intensity and cultural boundedness of prejudices and discrimination. Where to look for the answers? The answers to the moral, practical and political quandaries posed by prejudice, racism and discrimination must be sought not only in characteristics of individuals and groups, but also in 'characteristics of society that affect us all' (Becker, 1967, p. 239) and in the tension between democratic modes of domination and sympathy, control and compassion (Fassin, 2005).

The third principle is rooted in the dictum aptly formulated by Blumer: 'respect the nature of the empirical world and organize a methodological stance to reflect that respect' (1998 [1969], p. 60). In order to understand the characteristics of society and the tensions at the heart of modern democracies, social psychologists can make more use of intellectual practical-theoretical tools outside the discipline that can complement and provide a thorough and deeper understanding of transformation and social change. As critical theorists, social psychologists are well placed to open dialogues and explorations of the research practices and assumptions of sociologists, anthropologists and historians as they engage with the various meaning-making layers through which society is organized and reproduces itself, and as they describe the complexity of universalistic and particularistic presuppositions of modern (democratic) culture.

Structure of the book

In this book I put critical analysis to the test by exploring, and offering a commentary on, the complexity of anti-Roma prejudices in Europe. I contend that critical analysis may serve as a necessary conceptual and empirical bridge to understanding the many facets of anti-Roma discrimination, inequality and moral exclusion, including those that have immediate, as well as those that have pernicious and long-lasting effects.

In Chapter 1 the sketching of the contours of critical analysis in social psychology is accompanied by a discussion of the nature of the discourse directed at the Roma minority (and the wider phenomenon of Romaphobia) in Western and Eastern Europe as a prototypical example of extreme prejudice. The chapter argues that extreme prejudice is a culturally and ideologically situated phenomenon. Discursive analyses in Chapters 5, 6 and 7 will suggest that both lay and elite talk about the Roma minority in Western and Eastern Europe is more extreme than the conventional anti-alien, anti-immigrant prejudiced talk. It is more extreme because Roma are portrayed not merely as 'different', but rather as beyond moral acceptability. Text and talk about Roma employs a style that denies but, at the same time, also protects and reproduces negative or life-threatening conduct against them. Perceptions of what makes prejudice against Roma extreme tend to differ across situations and contexts. But, as I will be arguing, it is not just the content of discourse that makes prejudice extreme, but also the socio-psychological, political and material consequences that derive from it – alienation, displacement, loss of dignity and respect, dehumanization.

In Chapters 2, 3 and 4 I offer a synthesis and critical appraisal of the most important theoretical, empirical and methodological tenets of the social psychology of racism. These chapters are not intended as reviews of literature but rather as an intellectual background for refining and supplementing the narrative thread on anti-Roma prejudices opened up in Chapter 1, by highlighting the importance of researching the cultural reproduction of racism. Chapter 2 critically discusses some of the core tenets of researching stereotypes and the conceptual apparatus used to describe and explain the continuously changing nature of racism. I briefly trace the historical career of these notions (and their contemporary equivalents or reinterpretations) and assess their conceptual and empirical viability. I ask how useful these notions are for understanding the subtle, as well as the more direct and extreme manifestations of contemporary anti-Roma racism. How easy is it to distinguish between 'new' and 'old-fashioned' forms of racism when confronted with complex manifestations of prejudice? What is the meaning of 'prejudice' and 'discrimination' associated with the traditional vocabulary of 'stereotyping' and 'new racism'?

Chapter 3 discusses the classic perspective of the 'authoritarian personality' and exegesis, and more recent developments in personality research. In this chapter I ask: What is the contemporary value of the 'authoritarian personality'? What can still be learned from this approach? What aspects have been overrated or unjustly ignored? How is this perspective reinterpreted, completed, by contemporary researchers? I conclude the chapter with a discussion of two key limitations of the personality approach: (1) its inability to account for the historical specificity of prejudices and (2) its failure to explain the variability, existence and ideological force of different types of prejudices.

Chapter 4 explores the role of social categorization in social cognition and social identity approaches to understanding racism in society. In the first part of the chapter I focus on 'ambivalent sexism', implicit prejudice and 'collaborative' approaches on prejudice. I critically discuss social cognition's tendency to conceive of prejudices as relatively stable and common features of our inner mental universe that can be 'measured' with the help of standardized instruments, and predilection for the study of automatic processes of cognitive processing of information and not the specific content of prejudices associated with certain ethnic groups. In the second part of the chapter I engage with a critical reading of social identity theory (SIT) and self-categorization theory (SCT). I briefly evaluate the contribution of the minimal group paradigm, the importance attached to categorization in classic studies, as well as in recent developments related to social mobilization and social change, collective action and research on self-definition and multiple identities. The theoretical scaffolding of SIT and SCT starts from the idea that society is constructed and structured along the lines of discrete social categories in relations of power, status and prestige with one another. What are the critical implications of such a view for the study of racism? What does it allow us to 'see' and what does it obscure? What separates SIT and SCT from the social cognition perspective? I close the chapter with a discussion of both social cognition and social identity theories' difficulties with symbolic aspects of Roma identity, and issues of ethnic minority self-definition.

Chapters 5, 6 and 7 explore anti-Roma racism as discursive and morally exclusionary ideology. Chapter 5 is, for the most part, theoretical, whereas

Chapters 6 and 7 discuss empirical examples. In Chapter 5 I suggest that perspectives based on discourse analysis offer a more comprehensive response to some of the theoretical and empirical quandaries of conventional social psychologies of racism, although they are not themselves devoid of limitations. Here I show how discourse analysis can be a very useful tool for uncovering and documenting the ways in which prejudices are constructed and reproduced in and through discursive actions and drawing on the ideological repository of symbolic knowledge in society.

Chapter 6 focuses on constructions of moral transgression in lay and elite talk about the Roma. It shows how complaints about spatial transgressions and misconduct, the use of spatial and cleanliness metaphors, as well as various other discursive and cultural resources, are used to construct morally exclusionary representations of the Roma. In Chapter 7 I expand the argument of Chapter 6 by considering the links between delegitimization, dehumanization and moral exclusion of Roma.

The last chapter of the book (Chapter 8) advances the idea that the answers to the quandaries posed by the study of prejudices more generally and against the Roma, in particular, do not lie in identifying the similarities or differences that divide various schools of thought or models of social change. The answers must be sought in social scientific frameworks that propose and foster a deeper and more meaningful dimension of social and cultural analysis and critique. There is a need for a renewed social psychology of racism, one that can move beyond existing theoretical and empirical models that attempt to explain social and ideological processes and power relations in terms of internal psychological processes, or posit the inevitability and/or the universality of prejudice and racism, without taking into consideration the specific ways in which prejudices are formed and reproduced socially, their symbolic weight and their influence on different forms of social and political organization and social responses to social problems. Here, I return to the framework of critical analysis outlined in the first chapter and I offer it as a possible corrective and as a potentially productive way forward. I also return to the idea of prejudice as indignity and argue that the tragic fate of Roma in Europe comes from the realization that, to paraphrase Taylor (1994), *being* Roma stacks the cards against the achievement of one's dignity *as* Roma. The tensions at the heart of civilized and decent societies (Western and Eastern European democracies), which engender prejudices and exclusionary practices, continue to play a major part in stacking the cards against Roma achieving full dignity, worth, respect and recognition in a global world. Prejudiced, as well as tolerant, discourses are part and parcel of the argumentative 'texture' of these societies, and social psychologists cannot continue to write the psychology of racism and moral exclusion without understanding their lingering contradictions. The question that should preoccupy more social psychologists of racism is not only why the Roma are Europe's new scapegoats, but also what is the nature of the prejudices against them, how do these prejudices come to life, how are they accomplished, and sustained over time, and what are their social, ideological, moral and material consequences?

Notes

1 The notion of 'status' is described as an independent dimension that allows us to make inferences about the worth of others based on socially developed 'status beliefs' that include perceptions of competence and agentic capabilities, meritocracy, influence, biased expectations, and social perceptions of difference – see Cuddy *et al.* (2007) for a social psychological account and Ridgeway (2014) for a sociological account. When salient, status beliefs bias people's judgements of difference and inequality.

Chapter 1

From antipathy to indignity

A framework for critical analysis

'Why examine prejudice – still?' This is the question that a recent collection on the neuroscience of prejudice and intergroup relations poses to the educated reader (Derks *et al.*, 2013). As one would expect, framing an answer to this question starts with defining what prejudice is. The definition offered by the editors reproduces the most dominant insight in the social psychology of racism and intergroup relations (Dixon and Levine, 2012), the idea of prejudice as 'negative evaluation': 'prejudice denotes the tendency to evaluate or judge people negatively before we know them, merely because of their membership in a particular group or social category' (Derks *et al.*, 2013, p. 2). This definition of prejudice is accompanied by a description of two core characteristics of prejudice that make it a worthwhile object of analysis: its pervasiveness and its complexity. As the editors argue:

> prejudice is pervasive in the sense that it is of all times, is present in all cultures, and is directed toward all kinds of different groups in society. Prejudice is complex in that it involves explanatory factors at intrapersonal (e.g. biological), interpersonal, intergroup, and cultural levels.
>
> (Ibid.)

The pervasiveness and complexity of prejudice should not be dismissed out of hand. It is not my intention to do so. What I want to highlight is that a focus on the pervasiveness and complexity of prejudice does not tell us much about its particularity, and plural manifestations. The fact that prejudice is pervasive does not mean it takes the same form everywhere. The fact that prejudice can be described as a 'fact of life' (Dixon and Levine, 2012, p. 3), very much in line with Allport's conception of prejudice, is arguably not enough to understand its societal anchorage, distinctiveness and uniqueness in certain societies and conditions. Prejudice is complex not only in the way it is explained but perhaps, more importantly, in the way that it is, in certain conditions, deeply embedded in the social organization of societies and connected to structural factors such as education, poverty, employment and criminal justice. Arguably, to write about prejudice in general terms does not offer a solid and satisfactory foundation for understanding its contingent and societal complexity.[1] As Bar-Tal (2000) argues, 'social psychology cannot escape from dealing with larger societal systems if it desires to be *social* in the broad meaning of the term and to be relevant to real problems that preoccupy people in their social life' (p. 156, emphasis in original).

Other researchers, whilst taking seriously the complexity of prejudice, account for it in terms of 'responses to specific social and historical circumstances' (Duckitt, 2013, p. 29). Duckitt (2013) argues that 'important changes in the historical context have begun to make different questions about prejudice, and different kinds of prejudice, salient for social scientists' (p. 38). The upshot of this view is that prejudice is a 'much more complex and multidimensional construct, affective in nature, and expressing basic human motives activated by particular social and intergroup conditions' (ibid., p. 40). The appreciation of social and historical conditions of prejudice can be seen as a precursor to a broader appreciation of prejudice – not limited to antipathy and natural (cognitive) functioning – yet it still does not account fully for how to approach or address prejudices deeply embedded in the social organization of societies and connected to macro systems and structural factors.

Early social psychologies of prejudice concentrated on social issues, social problems, of specific societies (e.g. Myrdal, 1996 [1944]) (where, interestingly, but relevantly, prejudice was only one aspect of analysis). Although they contained the seeds of universal and generalizable lessons, these analyses were very much located in and spoke to specific socio-historical and cultural contexts, and treated prejudice not just as a matter of fact (of life) but as social problem. The 'problems' that Myrdal wrote about were concerning dilemmas, deeply anchored, deeply embedded, in socio-structural and historical factors of a particular society, the United States. In a similar vein, Pettigrew (2007) identifies advances in American black–white relations, but also structural barriers (employment, health, criminal justice, education, poverty) that further 'serious racial disparities'. Pettigrew concludes that American black–white relations continue to pose a series of problems for contemporary American society. He also argues that social problems demand multi-level and multi-disciplinary analysis.

In this chapter I argue that, for certain types of contemporary prejudices (such as the ones against the Roma in Europe), a return to prejudice as a social and structural problem may be what is needed to revitalize a social psychology of racism steeped in cognitive, affective and motivational assumptions. In the next sections I make the case for the uniqueness and distinctiveness of anti-Roma prejudices as both a historical, or what Allport called 'stubborn' prejudices, and a contemporary social problem for European societies. Historical as well as contemporary manifestations of these prejudices show that democratic and liberal values are sometimes not enough to erode (a history of) intolerance.

A democratic and liberal ethos can actually cultivate social practices, institutions, societal systems that, routinely, exclude a certain type of people – those who are perceived as inadequate, failures, according to the motivational and moral schemes of liberal democracies. In certain conditions, the liberal, progressive ethos of liberal democracies can succumb to dogmatism, to a stance that awards freedom of choice, freedom of movement, etc., to some but refuses it to others. The diversity and intensity of prejudices against the Roma in a liberal, democratic Europe (a Europe 'for all') points to the failures, and inherent contradictions, of a liberal, progressive ethos. Moreover, a focus on the diversity and intensity of prejudices against the Roma can provide a renewed source for social psychological reflection on its conceptual apparatus, theories and empirical approaches, and a return to researching prejudices as an integral part of socio-structural, cultural and political arrangements.

Prejudice as a social problem

European states (and Roma themselves) are faced with the challenge of what some authors call European anti-Gypsyism (Nicolae, 2009) or Romaphobia (Ljujic *et al.*, 2012).[2] The criminalization of Roma in Italy (Costi, 2010), Roma killings in Hungary (Tábori, 2009), their frequent evictions or relocations in France, the erection of walls separating communities in Slovakia and the various calls for and cases of sterilization of Roma in some European countries are only a few examples of deliberate attempts to remove the Roma minority from the domain of moral acceptability. Descriptions used by ordinary people or declarations of public figures that Roma are the 'scum of the earth', or that they 'are animals and behave like animals' (Tileagă, 2014), add to an unflattering image of present-day Europe, where, with extraordinary regularity, the Roma are seen as expendable.

Ordinary people, politicians and decision-makers seem to agree that the Roma are unlike any other European minority group. For some, like George Schöpflin (Hungarian Member of the European Parliament), the Roma's existence is 'absolutely dysfunctional, in total opposition to the tradition of the majority'. The mayor of Cholet (western France), Gilles Bourdouleix, defended himself against accusations that he told a group of Roma that 'maybe Hitler didn't kill enough of them', whereas the mayor of Nice (southern France), Christian Estrosi, called for all French mayors to follow his methods (24-hour surveillance of the Roma), and 'not surrender'. The Roma, as a 'problem group', as a social problem, is a quite familiar, historical trope in European private and public discourse (for illustrations, see Fraser, 1992; Okely, 1983). Characteristics such as their inability to adapt to 'civilized' life, their transgression of moral and spatial boundaries and the failure of integration efforts are aspects of a widespread contemporary diagnosis that presents Roma as deviant and transgressors of moral/civilized boundaries of European societies.

European societies are engaged now, more than ever before, in a dialogue about the moral status that should be assigned to the Roma. There is wide agreement amongst national and European policy-makers that the Roma present a *social problem* that requires a 'European' (read 'rational' and 'acceptable') solution. Europeans seem to agree on the *existence* of a social problem, but they disagree on the *moral nature* of the 'problem' that Roma pose. This creates a tension between the European creed of law, justice, security and freedom for all, humanistic and progressive ideals and concrete (European) practices that exclude, debase, degrade a definite category of people – the Roma.[3] This dilemma or tension is 'ordinarily invisible' (Opotow, 2011), and one of the crucial aims of any social psychological analysis is to make its implications visible and understandable, and to spell out its significance. In his seminal study of racism in America, Myrdal (1996 [1944]) provided perhaps the most cogent example of the significance of moral dilemmas. Myrdal constructs his argument around the perceived tension between 'the Creed of progress, liberty, equality, and humanitarianism' (vol. I, p. 80) and the reality of segregation. It is this very tension that turns (at least in Myrdal's eyes) a national problem (the 'Negro problem') into a *moral* problem. The 'American dilemma' of which Myrdal speaks in the title of his book is a moral dilemma, an attempt to reconcile the national conscience reflected in the American creed and the 'reality' (and practices) of oppression and unequal intergroup relations. Prejudice as a social problem and moral dilemma is not something you measure (in the way you can measure 'attitudinal negativity' using a questionnaire). It is a challenge; not psychological, but societal.

The continuum of attitudinal positions and practices towards the Roma covers a very diverse range of shades and nuances – tolerant, compassionate, paternalistic, conflictual, eliminationist and genocidal. Common perceptions of Roma's parasitic existence and subhumanity (Petrova, 2003; Sibley, 1992, 1995) coexist with benevolent and paternalistic attitudes. These attitudes and practices span the political spectrum (Hockenos, 1993; Tileagă, 2005). In a recent interview about the treatment of Roma in France and Italy, Jacques Delors (former President of the European Commission) expressed the deep ambivalence of Europeans towards the Roma:

> the way that the Roma are treated in France and Italy is no less scandalous. Of course, the Roma cannot go just anywhere but to conclude from that that it is acceptable to destroy the places where they live and force them to return to Romania or Bulgaria is scandalous.
>
> (Delors, 2011)

So, according to Delors, it is immoral (but perhaps not racist) to displace or destroy Roma camps, but the fact remains – 'the Roma cannot go just anywhere'. Delors' position can perhaps be better described by what Norman

(2004) calls the 'ambiguity of solidarity'. In a study conducted in Sweden, Norman charts the different reactions to the establishment of a refugee camp in the town of Gruvbo. She shows how the various debates around the refugee camp triggered a wide range of responses – from 'the greatest hostility to a tolerant indifference or a certain compassion' (ibid., p. 211). The continuum of responses reflects a tension between the central precepts of Swedish legislation (equality, fairness and solidarity) and a social reality (and beliefs) that may not conform to such ideals.[4] Another example is offered by the recent Norwegian debate (triggered by the visible presence of Roma 'beggars') on whether to declare begging an illegal public practice. Whereas some towns and cities were prepared to introduce a zero-tolerance policy, the Norwegian town of Kristiansand voted in one of its recent council meetings to instal toilet and shower facilities for the town's 'beggars'. In France, in 2012, whilst talking about the Roma 'problem', the then Interior Minister Manuel Valls argued that his country 'could not welcome all the wretched of the earth'. He also argued that France was undergoing a 'crisis of authority', and that (national) security was not a right- or left-wing issue, but 'a value of the Republic'.

The issue of European extracommunitarian and intracommunitarian migration provides a more recent illustration of the tensions and ambiguities of solidarity. French anthropologist Fassin (2005) describes the inherent tension of French political programmes on immigration by recounting the fate of the former immigration centre of Sangatte, near Calais. Fassin uses the example of Sangatte to show how political decisions, and their practical, material and human consequences, contain tensions and seemingly contradictory repertoires: order and sympathy, repression and compassion. He notes how, before its closure, the centre was described as a 'focal point for human rights grievances' but also as a 'potential menace to the public order' (ibid., p. 364). The argument for its closure was based on the idea that the centre 'was a magnet for illegal immigration, and ... shameful for a modern democracy to allow such an institution to persist' (ibid.). The carefully crafted argument appeals to seemingly contradictory social values: on the one hand, a desire for order supported by pragmatism, and on the other hand, a desire for sympathy sustained by humanitarian values.[5]

What these examples show is that solidarity, justice and fair treatment are not guaranteed by abstract ideals enshrined in national constitutions; they are 'ambiguous', *conditional* and susceptible to the influence of lay and political currents of opinion. In the public sphere, solidarity, justice and fair treatment can turn into a disputed value. What these examples also show is that liberal democracies are complex mechanisms of domination as well as empowerment (Fassin, 2005). In the discourse of the elite (and lay members of society), familiar tropes of toughness are mingled with reasonableness, order/pragmatism is mingled with sympathy. This discourse is a social product of democracies; it originates from (and feeds back into) 'the cultural schemes of the society (or societies) in which historical action unfolds' (Sahlins, 2004, p. 292).

The Roma in Europe are perceived as the return of the unruly body, a collective that embodies *partial society*, whose rules, norms, behaviours do not square with the existing 'cultural schemes' of European societies. The creeds, the values, of liberal democracies embody the cultural *totality* of their cultural schemes. The cultural totality of liberal democracies is the background for the creation of what Boltanski and Thévenot (2006 [1991]) call 'tests' of worth. Liberal democracies are political totalities that do not tolerate partial societies, or 'communities that take themselves as society' (Taguieff, 1987, p. 484). The democratic ideal represented by the nation-state is that of the organic community. On the outskirts of European towns, the Roma construct partial societies, which are systematically destroyed by civil authorities. In theory, democracy posits that there is not a legitimate basis for a hierarchy of social groups, as they share the same rights in the human condition. In practice, democracy is intolerant to anything (procedures, rules, norms, ways of being in the world) that does not stand 'solid behind a reality that is all of one piece' (Boltanski, 2011, p. 154).

A framework for critical analysis

Researching the 'ordinarily invisible' dilemma or tension between the European creed of law, justice, security and freedom for all, humanistic and progressive ideals, and concrete (European) practices that exclude, degrade, humiliate the Roma, requires a distinctive framework – what I would like to call 'critical analysis'. As noted in the Introduction to this book, 'critical analysis' is not a version of more established critical approaches to the study of racism (although one can identify areas of overlap and subtle affinities), but rather an attempt to bolster a critical agenda by imbuing social psychological theory with a sociological and anthropological texture. By 'critical' I mean the potential of working with and within frameworks that conceive prejudice, racism and discrimination as a social and cultural system, firmly lodged in (and influenced by) the historic and current democratic societal (discursive, material, political, legal) orders. The primary aim of a critical analysis of racism is to understand the operative social practices and societal principles that span societal orders and regulate processes of inclusion and exclusion, the argumentative spaces they generate, the justificatory rhetoric that accounts for their continuous existence or resistance to them, and potential contradictions between declarations of faith and actual treatment of people.

Critical analysis in social psychology can offer grounds for a systematic social and moral critique of society rather than start (and end) with the belief 'that there is only one program which is directed toward all the good in the world' (Myrdal, 1996 [1944], p. 1061). Quite the contrary, it needs to be able to critique vigorously that position. The aim of critical analysis is to refine and broaden the current focus of the social psychology of racism. Insights from some of the most dynamic currents in anthropology, social theory and sociology (Boltanski, 2011, 2012; Fassin, 2005, 2008; Wacquant, 2008) can reinvigorate and reorient a renewed social psychology of racism. Empirical and conceptual grounding (and elaboration) can be achieved with the help of kindred fields. By turning to sociology, social theory and anthropology (and history of social and intergroup relations, more generally), the social psychology of racism can address both the issue of 'general laws' that 'deal with the relation between possible conditions and possible results' (Lewin, 1946 p. 36), and the issue of 'diagnosis' of specific situations. As Lewin argued, both types of research objectives are needed in social research.

Contemporary social psychologists of racism call for critical approaches to social change and intergroup relations where all 'heuristic avenues' are explored and more 'contextualist' perspectives are proposed (Dixon and Levine, 2012; Dixon *et al.*, 2013).

> In some contexts, we agree, the project of getting us to like one another may be crucial to producing social change. Under conditions of comparative equality between groups, for example, then the project of promoting 'peace, love and understanding' is often intrinsically valuable. In other conditions, however, prejudice may be an epiphenomenon that distracts us from the main causes of, and solutions to, problems such as race, class or gender discrimination. In still others, with an irony that is increasingly evidenced by research, prejudice reduction may actually become part of the problem that it is designed to solve, diminishing the extent to which members of historically disadvantaged groups acknowledge and challenge broader structures of social injustice.
>
> (Dixon *et al.*, 2013, p. 249)

I contend that the various puzzles identified by Dixon and colleagues are perhaps best resolved or at least considered with much clarity and depth by casting the net beyond the traditional boundaries of the discipline. Whereas some heuristic avenues in social psychology will continue to tread the beaten track of established approaches, critical analysis engages with and explores heuristic avenues that open a dialogue between social psychology and cognate disciplines.

Critical analysis is an attempt to give a more pronounced sociological, anthropological and historical flavour to both universalist and relativist social psychological analyses of prejudice, racism and discrimination.[6] According to a universalist philosophy, both subtle and blatant biases are considered universal features of the human condition (Fiske, 2002). The roots of prejudice (authoritarianism, social dominance, intergroup anxiety, threat and so on) are 'universals' that manifest themselves in every society (Sidanius and Pratto,

1999) and reflect the internal organization of personality (Mondak, 2010) or neural processes (Derks *et al.*, 2013). According to a relativist philosophy, both subtle and blatant biases are socio-communicative products. Racist discourse is argumentative discourse (Billig, 2002a; Tileagă, 2005, 2006, 2007; van Dijk, 1987), where shifts can be fluidly made between arguments of principle and practice, where liberal and illiberal tropes are used for potentially racist effect or to justify and legitimate inequality, unfair treatment and exclusion (Wetherell and Potter, 1992). People are careful to inoculate themselves against bias and disclaim prejudice, either by constructing their views as rationally arrived at (Edwards, 2003), or by finding reasons with a basis in the world rather than their own subjectivity (Augoustinos and Every, 2010; Tileagă, 2005).

Critical analysis complements universalist and relativist insights with insights from disciplines that have developed conceptual and methodological tools for critically appraising and describing the societal processes by which societies (democracies) design, promote and justify their own social and ethical orders. Although both universalist and relativist approaches have developed platforms for social justice and fighting inequality, their current forms and assumptions limit their critical potential. I discuss some of these limitations in subsequent chapters.

A critical analysis of racism takes the form of an integrated, holistic analysis of society and its presuppositions, including the power (and ability) to offend, degrade or transform/modify the worth of individuals and communities, with, but also, more importantly, without the presence of deliberate hatred. A critical analysis of racism would take into account the 'life-space' (Moscovici, 2011) of both extreme and subtler prejudices: their channels of reproduction, their sources and audiences, their composition, as well as their intersections, their societal expressions and contradictions.

Contemporary exclusionary and discriminatory practices of liberal democracies do not take the form of 'autistic hostility' (Newcomb, 1947), but rather, flexibly, combine a desire for order and compassion couched in a language of respectability. In order to address this quandary, social psychologists need to work with a conception of society (and democracy) that would help them define more precisely the contours of societal mechanisms of inclusion and exclusion, the societal mechanisms of assigning, transforming or altering people's worth and dignity.

Critical analysis opens the way for a meaningful, and renewed, social psychology of racism that can establish itself more as a sociology and anthropology, rather than a psychology, of modern democratic culture. This is in line with furthering the project of social psychology as an 'anthropology of modern culture' (Moscovici, 1972). This book assesses the value and possibility of such a project by exploring tragic fate of the Roma minority in Western and Eastern Europe.

Critical analysis rests on three central hermeneutic principles with roots in critical sociology and moral anthropology. The first two are conceptual. The third takes the form of a methodological suggestion.

The first principle refers to how individuals, groups and communities construct specific cultures, practices and actions, and act on themselves and others, thus recognizing each other's moral worth (Boltanski and Thévenot, 2006 [1991]). The worthy are 'those who embody the collective, represent the others and serve to express the general will' (Boltanski, 2012, p. 15). The unworthy are disruptive of the general will, they lack the strength of affiliation and solidarity that the worthy possess as a matter of fact. Democratic societies define forms of worth, respect and dignity that circumscribe private and public spheres (education, politics, health, law and justice, etc.). Within each of these public spheres, various individual, group and community justifications provide people with different degrees and intensities of worth. What makes a society a democracy is that it is a polity, tacitly or explicitly attending to a (pecking) 'order of worths' on the basis of which 'the relative worth of the beings present can be established' (ibid., p. 47).

For instance, what social psychologists call delegitimization (and its extreme form, dehumanization), whether described as psychological (Haslam and Loughnan, 2012; Leyens *et al.*, 2003) or discursive (Tileagă, 2007), is, in practice, the process of having one's worth weighed and transformed within societies' moral schemes. Whereas 'normal persons must thus agree to see their own worth vary' (Boltanski, 2012, p. 49), aliens, foreigners, refugees, minorities must agree to have their own worth modified by others, or, in extreme cases, taken away from them. Injustice and intolerance are enacted whenever the relative worth of people is not taken into account, and when the existing, legitimate order or regime of worth in a society offers the premises for the social and moral exclusion of people without the possibility of retort.

The second principle is tied to the idea that democracy embodies modes of domination, as well as empowerment/sympathy (Fassin, 2005). Although universal respect for human dignity is one of the fundamental features of democratic society (Misztal, 2012), nation-states create their own cultural politics and policies for dealing with otherness that alter the dignity of people. In liberal democracies, the various channels of reproduction of tolerance and intolerance (individual, institutional, legal, etc.) underpin cultural politics and policies that vacillate between a desire for order and sympathy, control and pity (Fassin, 2005). Critical analysis based on this principle can address the key challenges of the social psychology of racism: researching prejudice and racism as an aspect of collective life and collective definition by offering a deeper understanding of the collective social conditions that make both tolerance and intolerance possible (Tileagă, 2014).

The third principle is entrenched in the dictum aptly formulated by Blumer: 'respect the nature of the empirical world and organize a methodological stance to reflect that respect' (1998 [1969], p. 60). A corollary of this is that methods (and concepts) should emerge as a concentration on 'public affairs', on public problems, not for their own sake (Jahoda, 1982; Jahoda *et al.*, 1971). As Condor argues, 'from its inception, the social psychology of prejudice embraced modernist fantasies that the systematic application of scientific method could offer utopian solutions to societal problems of social inequality and conflict' (2006, p. 8). Interpretations are validated through or by the method from which they emerged. Theory offers support to this type of validation. Nothing else, apart from the methodological apparatus itself, can invalidate claims and interpretations. Social issues, 'public affairs', may inform the operationalization and methodological set-up but they play virtually no part in validating results and interpretations arising from it. Researching public affairs forces researchers to refrain from building a priori models, classifications, etc., and validity tests of the object under investigation, and work with data generated *in* and *by* cultural spheres. One major consequence of this would be the extension of social psychology's sources of data, not limited to the conventions of positivist and relativist approaches. Data would be a product of practice, not necessarily shaped by researchers to suit a particular approach, and created with the aim to make some aspect of social reality more visible, to support a culturally located account of a particular practice or aspect of social reality.

The social psychology of racism cannot simply concern itself with moral issues in the laboratory or in social interaction. It needs to confront insights from these settings in what ethnographers and anthropologists call 'field situations' and what social action researchers call 'field experiments in social change' (Lewin, 1946, p. 36). The aim is to render visible, and clarify, moral issues in their cultural, historical and practical contexts. For instance, field experiments in prejudice reduction show that research findings can emerge not just as a matter of researcher-led design but also out of 'the distractions, social interactions, and emotional reactions of a real-world setting' (Paluck, 2009, p. 583). Respecting the nature of the empirical world suggests that research would proceed and progress incrementally, iteratively, reflexively, through various social, cultural and political 'sites', which throw into the mix various valuations, positions, ambiguities. The trajectories of research projects would be 'mobile' and 'multisited', with analytic developments discovered along the way rather than a matter of design (cf. Marcus, 1998).

As Myrdal himself has made it clear in his analysis of American racism, contrived data is 'never enough for posing the practical problems concerning what is right, just, desirable and advisable' (1996 [1944], p. 1059). Naturally occurring data (texts, public debates, observational and behavioural data) sourced in the complex social imaginary of societies can be a potent way into understanding the various meaning-making layers through which both tolerance and intolerance are organized and operate in society. By respecting the nature of the empirical world, it is perfectly reasonable and possible to construct integrated theory 'with one eye to the realities of the context and the other to the generalities of theory' (Paluck, 2009, p. 584). Whether we are using semi-structured interviews, experimental designs, surveys, qualitative or quantitative analyses of public texts, we need to consider planned and explicit questions as well as open 'possibilities' and 'unintended consequences' in the research process (Carrithers, 2005) and be prepared to 'explore questions overtly present but also questions which remain covert or unformulated' (Fassin, 2008, p. 341).

I will come back to these principles and I will expand on them, and weave them into the argument, throughout the chapters of the book.

From antipathy to indignity

I could have reasonably chosen to frame the issue of the Roma's tragic predicament in Europe simply in terms of 'negative evaluation', irrationality, hostility or antipathy. I could have followed closely Allport's dictum: 'whatever our values may be prejudice is *a fact of mental organization* and *a mode of mental functioning*' (Allport, 1950, p. 4, emphasis in original). Allport devoted himself to considering prejudice as a natural human phenomenon, a by-product of categorical, natural thinking. According to him, 'erroneous generalization and hostility – are natural and common capacities of the human mind' (Allport, 1954, p. 17). Allport's exegesis and research programmes that sprang out of it (for illustrations and reviews, see Brown, 2010; Dovidio *et al.*, 2005) have advanced and unpacked the significance of Allport's meta-theory – 'thinking ill of others without sufficient warrant', the irrational, false, unjustified, negative evaluation of others.

As Reynolds *et al.* note, when social psychologists define prejudice as 'irrational' and 'unjustifiable' they are embedding an 'explanation for prejudice in its definition – "faulty and flawed" psychology' (2012, p. 49). Yet, the more I looked into (and realized) the complexity of European contemporary prejudices against the Roma, the more I realized that a different story was being told by the Roma themselves and other societal actors. And that story did not have much to do with a 'faulty' and 'flawed' individual psychology, or simply with unadulterated hostility or antipathy. Although it was undeniable that hostility, antipathy, towards the Roma was a key aspect of understanding the nature of prejudices against the Roma, it could only offer a specific and partial vantage point. If one was to consider hostility and antipathy (or what social psychologists would call 'attitudinal negativity') as the only problem one would be narrowing the scope of social psychological explorations.

Social psychologists have tried to qualify Allport's emphasis on negative evaluation by drawing attention to the role of both negative and positive attitudes or feelings about a person or a particular group in the production and reproduction of prejudice. For instance, Jones (1997) defines prejudice as a 'positive or negative attitude, judgment or feeling about a person'

(p. 10). More recently, research on gender discrimination and the notion of 'ambivalent sexism' points to the role of favourable attitudes towards women that can reproduce women's subordination (Glick and Fiske, 2001; Rudman, 2005). Jackman has argued against the notion of irrational hostility by noting that processes such as 'discrimination and violence are driven by self-interested, rational, political motives. The central motivator for dominant groups in unequal social relations is not hatred, but the desire to control' (2005, pp. 89–90). The idea underpinning this is that 'indiscriminate hostility is too incendiary to be effective. By contrast, *positive* beliefs and feelings – when offered on a conditional basis – have an unrivaled potency' (ibid., p. 90, emphasis in original). Other researchers point to the functional role of prejudicial attitudes. Jost and Hamilton argue that 'the specific contents of stereotypes and their prejudicial flavor are best accounted for in terms of social and cultural functions that these attitudes serve' (2005, p. 210). More recently, Dixon and Levine argue that racist language retains its ability to offend without the presence of deliberate hatred. As they argue, 'ideological process need not operate via the attribution of uniformly negative qualities to others. Nor, indeed, is it necessarily accompanied by expressions of unadulterated hostility' (Dixon and Levine, 2012, p. 311; see also Dixon *et al.*, 2012).

Other researchers have replaced Allport's negative evaluation metatheory with a new metatheory based on the importance of group membership. According to this view, 'prejudice is bound up with the dynamics of ongoing intergroup relations, and the way that people make sense of these relations and form a shared collective view of their social world' (Reynolds *et al.* 2012, pp. 49–50). Prejudice flows not from the psychology of individuals, but from social identities and social/political ideologies that are associated with these (Turner and Reynolds, 2003). Another important shift away from Allport's ontology was marked by approaches to prejudiced cognition that aim to restore 'agency and sociality to the prejudiced subject' (Durrheim, 2012, p. 196). The various attempts to research 'prejudice in the wild' through the perspective of distributed or collaborative cognition (Condor and Figgou, 2012) have documented the subtle role that social interactions play in the expression of various forms of prejudice. In everyday conversations, prejudices 'are gestured in forms of expression in which they are simultaneously revealed and hidden' (Durrheim, 2012, p. 194).

Discursive psychologists have also moved away from Allport's emphasis on categorization and inner cognitive processes by emphasizing the role of discourse in the reproduction of racism (Tileagă, 2005, 2007; Wetherell and Potter, 1992). Discursive psychologists have shown that there is more to understanding prejudice than considering its purported immutable and irrational quality. Prejudice is context-bound, shifting with many situations, working on many fronts and multiple manifestations. I discuss the implications of these shifts for understanding anti-Roma prejudices in Chapters 5, 6 and 7.

In a nutshell, Allport's critical exegesis has tried to do justice to the variety and complexity of forms that prejudice(s) can take by shifting the focus away from negative evaluation and irrationality. As I argue in subsequent chapters, a further shift is needed – from prejudice as antipathy to prejudice as harm inflicted by indignity. I have discussed in the Introduction the broad parameters of such a conception. Going beyond prejudice as negative evaluation can reveal the breadth and depth of paradoxes lodged at the heart of the social expression of prejudice in liberal democracies. Social psychologists continue to look for the nature of and remedies for prejudice in the psychological make-up of individuals, groups and collectives, instead of taking seriously its cultural, societal and moral paradoxes, where progressive and benevolent attitudes mingle with conservative and discriminatory actions, and where sympathy mingles with resentment and contempt (Jackman, 2005). One cannot 'dethrone hostility', as some authors have called for (cf. Jackman, 2005), without extending the definition of prejudice to include societal effects such as indignity, and without understanding the nature of collective definitions of common social experience that impact on how we define dignity, respect and worth as grounds for deciding who is included or excluded from the scope of justice and fair treatment.

Social psychologists are guided less by social problems, social issues and public affairs, and as a consequence they have been less concerned with societal dynamics or processes that make reference to societal paradoxes and unintended consequences of the 'prejudice problematic'. It is perhaps fair to say, following Condor and Figgou (2012, p. 202), that

> researchers have adapted their understanding of prejudice to capitalize upon changing social psychological fashions, interests and technological developments ... Researchers have been able to customize the prejudice problematic to enable them to employ almost every technique in the toolbox of social psychological methods.

I argue that the diversity and intensity of prejudices against the Roma can provide a renewed source for social psychological reflection on theory and method. It is increasingly clear that hostility and antipathy do not operate independently of other societal aspects; neglect, isolation, marginalization also play a role. The majority of commentators point not only to the pernicious effects of racism but also to the role of social and economic conditions in Europe. For instance, the American financier George Soros writes about a 'Roma problem in Europe', which, according to him, is getting worse. He argues that 'both the problem and its worsening reflect a toxic combination of deep-seated hostility and persistent neglect' (Soros, 2013). Kalman Mizsei, the chair of the board of the Making the Most of EU Funds for Roma programme of the Open Society Foundations, contends that 'isolation of and discrimination against Roma not only undermines European values; it threatens to unravel the social fabric in Europe's new democracies' (Mizsei, 2012).

For most Europeans, the Roma continue to represent the epitome of foreignness. The Roma are perceived as unmeltable ethnic minorities (MacLaughlin, 1998), the inner enemy (Sigona, 2003), the alien next door (Bauman, 1990); they were historically (and still are) a 'problem' that needs a 'solution'. The Roma 'problem' is a social problem of an enlarged Europe. The determinants of this social problem may be objective or subjective, proximate or distal, minimized or intensified by social or institutional forces. At the same time, many of the determinants of this European social problem remain easy to miss or difficult to raise because 'they confront our values with a reality we would rather avoid' (Fassin, 2006, p. 3).

For centuries, the Roma were victims of a special kind of racism, one 'which juxtaposes nationalism and colonialism in such a way as to draw clear distinctions (and boundaries) between the "civilized native" and the "barbaric other"' (MacLaughlin, 1998, p. 1023). The current European project of managing diversity does not seem to find an appropriate place for Roma's (European) aspirations. Freedom of movement and settlement, the pillars and ultimate expression of democratic dignity in an enlarged Europe, is only conditionally offered, and in some cases outright refused, to the Roma. The current European project of managing diversity also shows how fragile human dignity is.

A social psychological framework that focuses on societal mechanisms of altering human worth and dignity is, arguably, more sensitive to what some scholars have described as Roma 'uniqueness'.[7] It can also prove to be more sensitive to moral issues and concerns that societies pose to themselves by developing ethnographies of social, cultural and political processes. Liberal democracies reflect and reproduce what American anthropologist Marshall Sahlins called a 'brave new anthropological world' (2004, p. 149) that parades 'subjects' and 'subjectivities', 'selves' and 'identities', 'relations'. Social psychologists should be able to engage with this 'new anthropological world' and describe how it frames the quandaries that democracies throw at themselves, especially those related to the moral inclusion and exclusion of people.

Notes

1 It would be odd, for instance, to construct a rationale for researching the Holocaust in terms of the pervasiveness and complexity of prejudice more generally. Similarly, it would indeed be odd to construct a rationale for researching the nature of anti-Roma prejudices by alluding to the general pervasiveness and complexity of prejudice.

2 See Crowe (2008) for an overview of the situation of Roma in post-communist Eastern Europe, and Barany (2002) for a history of Eastern European Gypsies. For the Nazi persecution of Roma, see Kenrick and Puxon (2009). More recent

accounts on the fate of Roma in Europe can be found in a wealth of reports on Roma integration and the successes/failures of implementation of education, policing and public health policies (e.g. Open Society Institute, 2011) or in reports that chart the repeated failures of European countries to protect Roma from racist violence (e.g. Amnesty International, 2014).

3 The European creed (if indeed there is such a thing) reflects not only the contemporary values of the European project, the European 'conscience', but also historical and religious values that pre-date it.

4 Similarly, in a study with Finnish Roma activists, Nordberg (2006) identifies a tension between the universalist ideals of the Finnish welfare state and a felt sense of exclusion from (full) citizenship experienced by Roma activists. According to Nordberg, the same national culture that encourages Roma activism and citizenship aspirations also contains the seeds and mechanisms that stifle the practicality of achieving citizenship status.

5 The debates around multiculturalism in European societies point to similar dilemmas. First, how to expand the scope of democracy in order to sidestep what Wieviorka (1998) has called the 'tyranny' of both majorities and minorities. Second, how to apply multiculturalism as a general rule and effectively, without 'the risk of excluding some groups who could legitimately demand to benefit from it' (p. 901). An added tension at the heart of multiculturalism is that between the universal and the particular. 'Not all cultural particularisms', writes Wieviorka, 'are necessarily amenable to a multiculturalist policy, or wish to be shaped by it' (ibid.). Arguably, the failure of multiculturalism in Europe is a failure of resolving the tensions at the heart of multiculturalism.

6 On the histories of the two dominant philosophies in the social psychology of racism, see Durrheim (2014).

7 For instance, Barany points out that 'the uniqueness of the Gypsies lies in the fact that they are a transnational, nonterritorially based people who do not have a "home state" that can provide a haven or extend protection ... The Gypsies ... are unique in their homelessness a situation that, in important respects, explains their marginality as well as their relationship to the states of Europe and beyond' (1998, p. 143).

Chapter 2

Stereotypes, new racism and the changing nature of marginality in Europe

In the first chapter I introduced the main tenets of a framework for critical analysis in social psychology of racism. I have also argued that the diversity and intensity of prejudices against the Roma can provide a renewed source for social psychological reflection on theory and method, and conceptual apparatus. The first section of this chapter opens with an outline of the classical view on stereotypes. I then offer a sketch of modern approaches to stereotyping, before moving to outline and critique the 'new' or 'modern' racism research legacy. The final section of the chapter considers the case of a move beyond stereotypes and notions of 'new' racism in the context of the changing nature of marginality in Europe.

Stereotypes as traits and 'biased' attitudinal products

In the introduction to their paper on stereotypes in social psychology, Augoustinos and Walker (1998) argue that 'no other concept in social psychology has evoked so much ambivalence as that of stereotyping' (p. 629). Stereotypes portray a particular social group or category (being a woman, Italian or German) as homogeneous. Individuals in those categories are being reduced to the 'essential' characteristics isolated by the stereotype. As Brown (1995, p. 82) suggests,

> to stereotype someone is to attribute to that person some characteristics which are seen to be shared by all or most of his or her fellow group members. A stereotype is, in other words, an inference drawn from the assignment of a person to a particular category.

Social stereotypes exaggerate, isolate and homogenize traits held to be characteristic of particular categories. The roots of this early conception of stereotypes and stereotyping can be traced back to work of Walter Lippmann in cultural studies. Lippmann was the first author to make reference to stereotyping in its modern sense in his book *Public Opinion* (1922). His concern with stereotypes was not that of a psychologist, but of a scholar interested in the role of the media in the political process. He was predominantly interested in the political uses to which stereotypes (especially those propagated by the media) could be put. As Pickering (2001, p. 17) suggests, outside social psychology,

> he deserves credit for his serious re-evaluation of the liberal model of citizenship and his considered appraisal of some of the obstacles standing in the way of effective political democracy, particularly in relation to the role of the media in the political process. Media stereotyping was one of the specifically modern political problems which he dealt with in connection with this process.

Social psychologists have acknowledged Lippmann as the precursor of modern research on stereotypes and stereotyping, but they have not really paid much attention to the different ways in which he conceived stereotypes. Lippmann identified stereotyping as a serious problem in opinion formation and expression. He conceived stereotypes in two opposed ways (see Pickering, 2001 for a full account). On one hand, he emphasized a 'political' sense of stereotypes, viewing them as inadequate and biased, endorsing the interests of those who use them and as obstacles to rational thinking and impervious to change. On the other hand, he regarded stereotyping as a necessary mode of processing information, an inescapable way of creating order out of the 'great blooming, buzzing confusion of the outer world' (Lippmann, 1922, p. 81). In this, latter, 'psychological' sense, stereotypes are equated with our general ways of thinking and attempts to make sense of the world and social actors within it.

According to Lippmann, stereotypes also functioned as rationalisations to maintaining social standing and status. Lippmann seemed to be aware of the contradiction between the two ways of thinking about prejudice, although he did not offer a direct way of reconciling the two conceptions. According to his 'political' conception, stereotyping was seen as an endemic problem in (modern) societies. The aim of researching the role of the media in reinforcing existing 'pictures' in our heads was to think of and devise solutions for the dilemmas it posed. According to his 'psychological' conception, stereotyping was no longer a negative process, but rather one from which human beings could gain. As a complexity-reducing process, stereotyping was seen and described as a necessary and crucial ingredient for making sense of the world. Perhaps Lippmann's most important contribution to social psychology is not the often-quoted description of stereotypes as 'pictures in the head' but the intellectual platform he built for understanding the cultural anchoring of stereotypes. As Lippmann argues,

> in the great blooming, buzzing confusion of the outer world we pick out what our culture has already defined for us, and we tend to perceive what which we have picked out in the form stereotyped for us by our culture.
>
> (1922, p. 81)

Social psychologists developed Lippmann's psychological concern with stereotypical content, whilst underplaying the cultural and political consequences of stereotypes and stereotyping. Lippmann was not specifically concerned with traits ascribed to groups of people, yet most of the classic empirical studies in social psychology did concern themselves with such trait attributions, particularly to ethnic groups.

During the 1930s, a major interest was developing in the measurement of attitudes as a bridge between understanding culture and individual behaviour. With the pioneering studies of Katz and Braly (1933, 1935), who were principally concerned with national stereotypes, the study of individual attitudes and values held about racially stereotyped groups became of central concern.

Using checklist methodology, Katz and Braly (1933) asked Princeton University students to check traits they thought described ten national groups. Those traits of a particular group that gathered considerable consensus were seen as stereotypic of that group. For example, 78 per cent of subjects thought that Germans were scientific-minded, whereas 54 per cent thought that Turks were cruel. In a second study, Katz and Braly (1935) discovered that the rank order of preferences for groups rated was identical to the rankings in terms of the average desirability of the traits ascribed to those groups. The ascription of traits to groups reflected culturally derived stereotypes or images about people representing those groups.

The early studies of stereotyping were designed and used to explain the effects of culture on prejudice and discrimination. The stereotypes identified by Katz and Braly were not the outcome of individual experiences with people from diverse groups, but rather cultural, 'biased' attitudinal products, largely reflections of the culture in which respondents were living. As erroneous cultural images of other people, stereotypes were the basis of negative evaluations, which, in turn, justified discrimination.

Katz and Braly's pioneering work was the beginning of a long tradition of seeing stereotypes as sets of traits associated with groups, with implications for prejudice and discrimination. For example, Ashmore and Del Boca conceive stereotypes as 'a structured set of beliefs about the personal attributes of a group of people' (1979, p. 222). In a similar fashion, stereotypes have come to be defined as 'sets of traits attributed to social groups' (Stephan, 1985, p. 600), or 'a collection of associations that link a target group to a set of descriptive characteristics' (Gaertner and Dovidio, 1986, p. 81). Stereotypes were also described as essentially deficient and inaccurate, rigid and 'hasty' over-generalizations, yet, in certain conditions, rectifiable and subject to change.

From pathologies of cognition to natural mental representations

With the publication of *The Authoritarian Personality* (Adorno *et al.*, 1982 [1950]), stereotypes began to be considered manifestations of a general prejudiced attitude. Stereotypes were viewed less as pictures in people's heads, but more as pathologies of individual cognition. Their source was intra-individual, intra-psychic personality dynamics and (pre)dispositions, which were thought to predict prejudice and discriminatory behaviour. As pathologies of social cognition, stereotypes were seen as cognitive products that were rigidly held in order to protect against ambivalence and ambiguity. They were seen as fundamentally incorrect, dogmatic and derogatory generalizations about groups of people, irrational and flawed cognitive products of a certain category of people (or a certain type of personality) nurtured in a very specific (highly hierarchical and conformist) type of society. I discuss the implications of this position and the social psychology of personality and disposition, and Adorno *et al.*'s exegesis and critique, in more detail in the next chapter.

In *The Nature of Prejudice*, Allport (1954) took a different approach. Although he did not discount the danger posed by authoritarianism, he devoted himself to considering prejudice as a natural human phenomenon, a by-product of categorical, natural thinking and information processing.

He offered a detailed discussion of the various cognitive factors involved in prejudice and stereotyping. Unlike Adorno *et al.*, Allport's concern was with the 'average' individual, the individual 'perceiver', and the basic cognitive propensity to place things and people into categories. Allport distinguished between categorization as a 'rational' and normal process and irrational stereotyping. Stereotypes, as an outcome of categorization, only turn to prejudice when new knowledge does not lead to revision and change. Allport's move in distinguishing between a 'normal' process of categorization and irrational stereotyping works at the same time to normalize, naturalize, but also pathologize prejudice. I will return to categorization, namely social categorization and its role in identity processes, in Chapter 4.

As noted in Chapter 1, Allport sets the scene for defining prejudice as a negative attitude towards members of particular groups, as 'antipathy based upon a faulty and inflexible generalization' (Allport, 1954, p. 9) serving an 'irrational function' (Ackerman and Jahoda, 1950). In this context, stereotypes were considered rigid, faulty and inflexible ways of thinking about individuals and groups (cf. Allport, 1954; Stroebe and Insko, 1989).

One other important historical, but also theoretical, landmark that accounted for turning stereotypes and stereotyping into a cognitive notion was the work of Henri Tajfel on the cognitive aspects of prejudice – his classic article 'Cognitive aspects of prejudice', originally published in 1969 (which also features as a key chapter in Tajfel's *Human Groups and Social Categories* (1981)). Tajfel highlighted the 'importance of the adaptive cognitive functioning ... in the causation of prejudice' (1981a, p. 141). Tajfel considered that general cognitive processes cannot be neglected if one wants to study the formation, diffusion and functioning of social stereotypes (Tajfel, 1981b). Understanding 'the cognitive "mechanics" of stereotypes is essential for their full and adequate analysis' (Tajfel, 1981a, p. 145), he argued. However, he also wondered 'whether such a study is all that is needed' (ibid.).

With the development and increased influenced of cognitive psychology, stereotypes and stereotyping were turned into a completely cognitive notion (Fiske and Taylor, 1991). Stereotypes were described as cognitive mental representations of groups and individuals based on 'normal' information-processing mechanisms and 'natural' categorization process, with a stable internal organization (Hamilton and Trolier, 1986). Stereotypes were seen 'as relatively mundane inhabitants of our mental world ... shortcuts the mind uses to simplify and understand the social world' (Locke and Johnston, 2001, p. 109).

Early research on category 'accessibility' and 'fit' (Campbell, 1958), research on object classification and categorization (Cantor and Mischel, 1979), cross-categorization research (Deschamps and Doise, 1978) or studies on the schematic organization of stereotypic knowledge (Fiske and Taylor, 1991) have solidified the belief that the content of people's cognitions about social groups is governed by the stable cognitive organization and (relatively automatic) functioning (and activation) of associations that link categories with presumed characteristics of individuals or groups. Countless times research has demonstrated the importance of processes of stereotype activation and use (e.g. Devine, 1989, 1995; Greenwald and Banaji, 1995). Although the mere possession of stereotypes need not inevitably lead to prejudice (see Devine, 1989, 1995), all (good) people carry 'hidden biases' (Banaji and Greenwald, 2013). According to Banaji and Greenwald, social groups (the world around us) and our minds interact and influence us without our awareness or conscious control. We all carry stereotypes of groups in society in our mind and we are unaware when and how these stereotypes have been activated, or how they influence our behaviour towards others.

Stereotypes and social structure

Stereotypes are not only rooted in our cognitive make-up and natural information processing but also in social expectations and structural relations between groups.

Researchers have also demonstrated that stereotypes can function as social 'hypotheses' for which we seek (social) support by turning to social context. For example, Darley and Gross (1983) have found that social class stereotypes can influence people's judgements of children's academic performance. Stereotypes generate behavioural expectancies, which can function as self-fulfilling prophecies (Rosenthal and Jacobson, 1968). In our social reasoning, we are more inclined to look for social information that confirms our 'hypotheses', and tend to discount information that falsifies them (Leyens *et al.*, 1994). Stereotypes can 'bias' our attributions of groups (and group categories) (Duncan, 1976; Pettigrew, 1979) and social events (Tajfel, 1981b).

More recent studies shift the emphasis to understanding more about the content of stereotypes in terms of perceived competition (between groups) and perceived status. Stereotypes are seen as rooted in social structure, in perceptions of social stratification and structural relations between groups (Cuddy *et al.*, 2009). As Cuddy *et al.* (2009) argue, 'a group's stereotype follows from perceived status and competition with other groups. However, culture influences group status and perceived group competition. Hence, specific groups' stereotypes vary cross-culturally' (p. 26). The content of group stereotypes is derived from the interaction between two universal dimensions of social perception: warmth and competence. Social emotions such as admiration, contempt, envy and pity are mediated by attributions of competence or warmth.

Structural relations between groups – relative status and interdependence (competitive or cooperative) – determines the content of group stereotypes. Powerful or successful minorities are said to be subject to envious prejudice (these groups are stereotyped as highly competent, said to harbor hostile motives and have more ability and power). In this category one would include 'respected-but-disliked' groups such as Asians or Asian-Americans, or Jews, which are the targets of envious prejudice and ambivalent stereotyping. Low-status groups are stereotyped as incompetent (less ability and power) (see, for instance, pitying or paternalistic stereotyping/prejudice towards older people and traditional women). According to Glick (2005), it is 'precisely the perceived power of a group … that makes it likely to be scapegoated' (p. 254). Glick also argues that the 'choice of scapegoat' is primarily influenced by 'prior envious stereotyping … of groups that are viewed as having the power and intent to cause widespread harm' (ibid., p. 253).[1]

By emphasizing the importance of the perceived relative status of groups, the role of ambivalent stereotypes that 'typically do not contradict prejudice or reduce discrimination but reinforce unflattering stereotypes on the other dimension and justify unequal treatment' (Cuddy *et al.*, 2008, p. 68) and how different types of prejudice (paternalistic and envious) operate (Glick and Fiske, 2001), social psychologists are offering robust evidence in support of the broader idea embraced by sociologists that the perceived relative status of groups serves as an anchor for judgements of the *worthiness* of majority and minority social actors (Ridgeway, 2014). Yet, taking all these aspects into account does not necessarily predict how certain groups will be actually treated, and how certain groups may respond to direct or ambivalent stereotyping.

Although it is vital to consider social and structural relations between groups in society, issues of relative status and system justification, as foundations for the formation and reproduction of stereotypes, one also needs to thoroughly engage with how stereotypes are discursively constructed in everyday and elite communications for particular and context-dependent rhetorical ends. As Augoustinos and Walker put it, 'stereotypes are flexible and dynamic representations which are constructed in situ, within a specific relational context at a particular point in time' (1998, p. 635). It is especially when one contemplates the link between stereotypes and social structure/status-driven relations between groups that one needs to explore and understand the nature of stereotypes as discursive and rhetorical constructions that people use 'to do things', such as to blame, justify, exonerate, etc. Although social psychologists conceive of stereotyping as a psychological process steeped in cultural and socio-structural assumptions about relative status and worth of individuals, groups and communities, they do not also, specifically, explore the socio-communicative nature of this process. One cannot conceive of stereotypes and stereotyping without a complementary focus on language and communication. People's assumptions and descriptions of relative status, or worth, are not mobilized in a social vacuum. People's stereotypes (ambivalent or otherwise) that, arguably, derive from assumptions and descriptions of relative status, or worth, are tied to an argumentative context, and they are socially transmitted, and ratified, culturally. As I will be arguing in Chapters 6 and 7, the legitimation of status quo and unequal social relations is not the only function of stereotypes. If one takes seriously the idea that stereotypes are discursive and rhetorical constructions, cultural products of specific societies, then it perhaps makes sense to also explore how people use available cultural resources to evaluate the worth of others, and what people are trying to do and what effects they are trying to produce with their talk (Edwards, 1991; Tileagă, 2005; Wetherell and Potter, 1992).

The idea of stereotypes as cultural products and reflections of socio-structural relations between groups supports the idea that 'stereotypes are not in themselves a full explanation for rejection ... they play an important part in prejudice but are not the whole story' (Allport, 1954, p. 189). Prejudices that originate in cultural stereotypes take a variety of forms, and do not necessarily derive from negative evaluations but more from societal assumptions reproduced and communicated in specific social and cultural contexts. Also, as Billig argued, prejudices 'can be distinguished in terms of their intensity and ideological importance' (2002a, p. 177). Thus, it is important to consider stereotyping (and its ideological consequences) in relation to wider societal conditions and ideological climates of opinion.

'New' racisms and types of people

The existence and persistence of ambivalent, paternalistic stereotypes point to the changing nature of societal prejudices. They point to what anthropologist Albert Memmi calls the 'strange kind of tragic enigma associated with the problem of racism' (Memmi, 2000) – although no one wishes to see himself or herself as racist, racism persists! Although liberal democratic societies place different types of legal and institutional controls on direct, hostile, expressions of prejudice, racism persists in subtle, ambivalent, paternalistic forms.

Social psychologists have been at the forefront of documenting the changing manifestations of racism. Earlier work was based on the observation that prejudice was declining and that racial values and ways of talking that could be defended without embarrassment a hundred years ago were no longer socially acceptable. In 1954, Allport could bring some historical and empirical evidence to argue that stereotypes 'change in time'. He wrote about stereotypes 'weakening in mass media' and about the 'upswing in intercultural education' that 'may ... be having an effect on ethnic clichés in the minds of today's students' (p. 202). 'All in all', he argued, 'the younger generation may be less stereotype-ridden than the parent generation' (ibid.). Other social psychologists point out that these changes are only relative and could be seen only in relation to some groups but not others (Dovidio and Fazio, 1992). Billig warned social psychologists not to be complacent when considering the changing nature of racism. As he argued, just because one can observe changes in the frequency and content of ethnic stereotypes, it does not mean that 'the racial store of common-places has been declared locked until further notice' (Billig, 1996, p. 247). What it means is that 'detached from their old value, some racist images, beliefs, and even feelings may now travel under the protection of acceptable, and formerly contrary, values' (ibid.). As a consequence, it may be more reasonable to assume that, in certain conditions, changes in the frequency and content of ethnic stereotypes might be seen more as a sign of stereotypes adapting to 'the prevailing temper of prejudice' (Allport, 1954, p. 204) than an indication of an actual reduction of prejudices. In this context what matters more is describing the *manner* in which people are prejudiced, alongside describing the societal conditions under which stereotypes change and adapt to the 'prevailing temper of prejudice' in specific societies.

Modern social psychology has coined a plethora of terms to capture the diversity of 'racisms' that were considered to form the basis of different expressions of prejudice (for reviews, see Brown, 2010; Duckitt, 1992): 'symbolic racism' (Sears and Kinder, 1971), 'modern racism' (McConahay, 1982), 'ambivalent racism' (Katz and Hass, 1988; Katz *et al.*, 1986), 'aversive' and 'dominative' racism (Dovidio and Gaertner, 2004; Gaertner and Dovidio, 1977, 1986), 'blatant' and 'subtle' prejudice (Pettigrew and Meertens, 1995;

Pettigrew *et al.*, 1998). These were all notions designed to capture the particularities, and subtleties, of a changing 'racism'. For example, McConahay and Hough (1976), McConahay (1981, 1982) and Kinder and Sears (1981), looking at people who voice anti-black sentiments, were proposing a distinction between 'new racism' (which includes people who typically deny their own prejudices) and 'old-fashioned red-necked racism' (which includes people who unambiguously use and declare their adhesion to racial values).

The notion of 'modern racism' was applied in other intergroup contexts, such as race relations in South Africa (Duckitt, 1991), the United Kingdom (Brown, 1995) and Australia (Pedersen and Walker, 1997). In the United Kingdom, Reeves (1983), in his analysis of British racial discourse, observed a 'sanitization' of the discourse of legitimation, similar to the one identified by other researchers in other countries (cf. Essed, 1991).

As various researchers working within this framework have shown, 'modern racism' is expressed in covert ways, which avoid a direct appeal to racial values. Discourse analyses of talk about minorities have corroborated the main presuppositions of modern racism approaches. Van Dijk's (1984, 1987, 1993) discourse-analytic studies of racism share a similar pattern to that of the 'modern racism' studies. Racist sentiments are simultaneously expressed and denied. Similarly, Billig (1988, 1991), Billig *et al.* (1988) and Cochrane and Billig (1984) analyse occurrences of denials of prejudice as a preface to complaining about blacks and ethnic minorities and find the same expression and simultaneous denial of prejudice. In the context of New Zealand, a similar pattern was found in the discourse of white, middle-class New Zealanders talking of Maoris (Potter and Wetherell, 1988; Wetherell and Potter, 1992). In these studies prejudices are 'justified in terms of any value but a racial one' (Billig, 1996, p. 248), and 'liberal' values are used to justify dominance, inequality and the status quo (Tileagă, 2006; Wetherell and Potter, 1992).

The language of contemporary racism is flexible, ambivalent and contradictory; speakers are at pains to appear rational and reasonable when uttering prejudiced comments. Whereas modern racist approaches theorize a conflict between psychological motives or propensities and socially acceptable expressions, and, routinely, place this conflict within the individual, discourse analyses of racism focus on the actual, flexible use of argumentative, cultural and rhetorical resources that reproduce inequality in liberal, egalitarian societies. As Wetherell and Potter have put it, 'the conflict is not between a feeling and a value, between psychological drives and socially acceptable expressions or between emotions and politics, but between competing frameworks for articulating social, political and ethical questions' (1992, p. 197). In Chapter 5 I explore in more detail the contribution of discourse-analytic approaches to the changing discourse of racism and manifestations of racism. For now it will suffice to note that, although they draw upon different epistemologies, the mainstream social psychological analysis of 'modern' racism and discourse-analytic approaches to racism are both concerned with understanding how racist values and beliefs transform themselves in combination with 'liberal' principles of democracy and equality of rights and diverse political commonplaces.

But, whereas discourse-analytic studies consider language use, modern racism approaches are more interested in producing (and working with) human types and individual differences. McConahay (1986), for example, writes about three groups of people. First, there are those who are 'tolerant', who are said to experience 'low negative affect' towards blacks and hold strong values of equality and freedom for all (these are individuals who exhibit strong positive anti-racist reactions); second, there are those who fall into the 'ambivalent' category – who experience an internal conflict because they have moderately negative feelings towards blacks but also value equality; and finally, those whose strong negative feelings towards blacks override the influence of societal values of tolerance and equal treatment. It is McConahay's ambivalent category that is described by the label 'modern racism'. The conflict that facilitates the expression of 'modern racism' is a conflict between liberal values and anti-black sentiments. 'Modern racists' do not endorse wholeheartedly the traditional negative stereotypes nor do they agree with segregationist views, yet they promote a practice of resistance to change in the name of historical American values.

The notion of 'symbolic racism' (Sears, 1988; Sears and Kinder, 1971) is based on a similar assumption: that values, standards and group norms that are widely shared within a community (or group) can shape prejudice and the way it is expressed. Prejudice is a complex mix of social and cultural norms (including the norm against the expression of overt prejudice). Symbolic racism, as the more acceptable expression of social and cultural norms, supplants (the unacceptable) biological racism. As Kinder and Sanders argue, 'prejudice is expressed in the language of American individualism' (1996, p. 106). Although rooted in cognitive and emotional processes, and primary and secondary socialization, symbolic racism is grounded more in culture than in individual psychology. Symbolic racism tries to reconcile the values of the American creed and anti-minority sentiments.[2]

The distinction between 'subtle' and 'blatant' prejudice (Pettigrew and Meertens, 1995) mirrors the traditional one between 'modern' and 'old-fashioned' prejudice, and emphasizes the role of perceived cultural differences. The crux of blatant racism is an overt amplification of cultural differences between majorities and minorities, whereas the crux of subtle racism lies in expressing negative feelings towards minority groups, subtly and indirectly, and a limited offering of positive evaluations and feelings. More recently, Bonilla-Silva discusses the ideological consequences of a 'racism without racists'. He examines the ideology of colour-blind racism in the United States that has replaced the more extreme 'Jim Crow' racism as 'the ideological armor for a covert and institutionalized system in the post-civil rights era' (Bonilla-Silva, 2014, p. 3). He goes on to argue that 'this new ideology ...

aids in the maintenance of white privilege without fanfare, without naming those who it subjects and those who it rewards' (ibid., p. 4).

Diverse types of people populate this psychological world of modern, symbolic, colour-blind expressions of prejudices. The 'benevolent' or 'patronizing' racist, generally a well-meaning person but (unconsciously) motivated by beliefs in majority-group superiority (Jackman, 1994) mingles with the 'laissez-faire' (Bobo *et al.*, 1997) and 'color-blind' (Bonilla-Silva, 2014) racist. These (new) human types can blame minorities for their predicament, and as Dixon and colleagues have argued, they support an emergent ideology where 'widespread acceptance of the principles of equality, integration, and anti-discrimination is offset by widespread resistance to their concrete implementation' (2012, p. 12).

One of the crucial lessons of modern racism approaches is that, too often, the abstract liberalism of individualism and equal opportunities clashes with the practical aspirations of concrete liberalism. Appearing reasonable, unprejudiced, holds much more cultural weight than ensuring consistency between beliefs, values and actual behaviour. One also has to ask: How distinct are these 'new' forms from their 'old-fashioned' counterparts? How vital is the need to distinguish between human types? If one inspects closely the discourse of the so-called 'old racism' one can identify many of the qualified, 'reasonable' statements that are said to characterize 'new' racism. So, arguably, in order to look at the particularities of distinct or not-so-distinct forms of racism one has to consider actual discourses of prejudice, and the flexible uses of justifications, criticisms and other rhetorical resources. As Billig (1991) argues, 'the distinction between "old-fashioned" and "modern racism" may not always be a distinction in kind, but may reflect an ability to provide justifications, often *post hoc*, for views and positions' (p. 134). Yet, social psychologists concern themselves less with argumentative discourse and everyday justifications and more with designing sensitive enough instruments to capture the subtle, automatic, unintentional workings of needs, beliefs, motivations, feelings and (subtle) individual differences between people.[3] What I would like to call 'reasonable' prejudice presents serious challenges for social psychologists.

There is a tension at the heart of modern racist approaches – a desire to design subtler and subtler techniques to measure modern or 'reasonable' prejudice, and 'categorize' individuals into types, whilst not fully recognizing the inherent difficulties in measuring modern racism with reactive instruments like questionnaires, imagined scenarios or reaction-time tasks. Another tension lodged at the heart of modern racist approaches is that between the role of psychological factors within individuals (e.g. 'negative affect') as the primary, proximal cause and the role of social factors, socialization and cultural norms more generally. It is difficult to discern the full extent of the interaction between the two sets of factors when one is more inclined to frame the analysis in terms of individual differences.

Perhaps a more profitable way to resolve these two tensions of the modern racism problematic is to think of people as individuals caught in an 'ideological dilemma' (Billig *et al.*, 1988). On one hand, they do not want to be seen as prejudiced. On the other hand, they generally do not want to support anything that involves abandoning privileges or transfer of power, or threatens the status quo. In order to understand how prejudice can be achieved from a position of tolerance, one also needs to explore (particular) social, cultural, historical meanings of tolerance. As Allport (1954) argued, we tend to know more of prejudice than we know of tolerance. The notion of tolerance in liberal democratic societies presents its own dilemmas, tensions, contradictions. One of the problems with our current (democratic) conception of tolerance is that it implies that 'there is, indeed, something about minority groups which is to be tolerated' (Henwood, 1994, p. 45). It also presupposes 'a hierarchy rather than an equality of difference' (Henwood and Phoenix, 1996, p. 852).

The majority of insights on modern racism come to us from across the Atlantic. North America, with its long historical and contemporary history of inequality and tolerance, and its postindustrial social and political organization, has been (and continues to be) the background for an unparalleled source of social psychological insight. However, the democratic framework of liberal democracies in Western and Eastern Europe can also offer a similarly fertile ground from which a renewed analysis of modern racism would proceed. As I will be arguing in the remainder of this chapter, researching European minority groups like the Roma can point to some of the limitations of stereotyping and modern racism approaches and to more productive ways forward in the analysis of 'reasonable' prejudices.

Racism and the nature of marginality in contemporary Europe

It may be a truism today that 'modern' prejudices must uphold the values of tolerance and good understanding, even when expressing unequal views. As Tileagă (2005, 2006) has shown, unambiguous denunciations of (extreme) right-wing politics and policies are not necessarily followed by similarly unambiguous declarations of tolerance towards the Roma. Placing a safe moral distance between the self and right-wing politics and policies, building a self-assured distance between fair-mindedness and reasonableness on the one hand and bigotry on the other hand, can, nonetheless, open the way for the expression of both commonplace, and extreme, morally exclusionary prejudices. When one discovers that, when it comes to some groups (but not others), extreme prejudices span the whole of the political spectrum, there is less need to label or categorize individuals as certain types of people on a continuum of prejudiced attitudes, but a more stringent need to understand what kind of society, what type or form of social and institutional organization, what kind of history (of interethnic relations), facilitates these kinds of (special) prejudices.

An exclusive focus on negative stereotyping, and individual differences, cannot account for the persistence of what Allport aptly called 'stubborn prejudices' like anti-Semitism or, in this case, anti-Gypsyism. We know, from a variety of studies, that overt symbols of racism can be (and are routinely) forthrightly rejected, but not necessarily their societal and moral assumptions. We also know that this is one of the ways in which racism thrives in society. Yet, what we don't fully appreciate is how to make sense of this dilemma without associating it with one group of individuals (or type of person), without relying on identifying types of individual prejudices. We also need to include as a dimension of analysis the role played by liberal democracy itself, its cultural practices and institutions and its internal contradictions.

The analysis of Roma prejudices in Europe in this book could have followed the contours, and assumptions, of existing modern racist approaches. For instance, following McConahay, one could have distinguished between different types of individuals: 'tolerant' individuals (those who will experience 'low negative affect' towards the Roma and who will hold strong values of equality of treatment for all); 'ambivalent' individuals (those who will experience an internal conflict because they have moderately negative feelings towards the Roma but also value equality); and finally, 'prejudiced' individuals (those whose strong negative feelings towards the Roma outweigh the influence of societal values of tolerance and equal treatment). McConahay's description of different types of people (and prejudices) is taken to a different level by social cognition researchers interested more in the mental characteristics of subtle prejudices (cf. Fiske and Molm, 2010). What McConahay described as ambivalent prejudice is described by Fiske and Molm as the 'vast middle' between two opposing margins of the spectrum: on the one hand, blatant prejudice, 'hot-blooded and bloody-minded, coming from perceived threat' (p. 343); and on the other hand, 'pure egalitarian orientations', 'open, liberal, and humanitarian, coming from felt security and values' (ibid.). The vast middle is that of 'subtle prejudice', which is described as 'cool, calm, and collective, mostly indirect and norm-driven'. As Fiske and Molm go on to argue, 'even well-intentioned people are … influenced by the culture's prejudiced portrayals, as well as by culture's anti-prejudice norms. The internal conflict drives people's biases into more subtle forms' (ibid.). Moreover, subtle prejudice, 'in all its guises … predicts everyday discrimination: uncomfortable encounters, avoidance, self-fulfilling prophecies, and ingroup-favoring decisions in voting, housing, education, and employment' (ibid., p. 344).[4]

If one were to focus solely on the modern and old-fashioned racists in McConahay's description one would miss the variety and forms of other prejudices shared by those who declare themselves 'tolerant', those who, seemingly, do not experience a conflict between their liberal values and their anti-Roma sentiments. One would also miss out on a fuller understanding of the societal *nature* of prejudices against the Roma more generally. Equally, if one were to focus solely on the 'vast middle' of Fiske and Molm's model, one would miss the variety and flexible nature of blatant and egalitarian prejudices against the Roma. The 'pure egalitarian orientations' are perhaps as important as 'hot-blooded' bigotry, and maybe more important than the subtle prejudices in the middle.

Researching subtle prejudices has become the new norm in the social psychology of prejudice and racism. Because subtle prejudices are seen to pose more of a theoretical and methodological challenge they are presented as universal prototypical prejudices in contemporary societies. What other researchers have called 'benign bigotry' is the new target of social psychological theorizing – those prejudices that are 'automatic, covert, often unconscious, unintentional, and sometimes undetectable by the target' (Anderson, 2009, p. 4).

Nier and Gaertner (2012) argue that 'there is indeed a predictable relationship between implicit measures of subtle bias and discriminatory conduct' (p. 213).[5] Even when one moves from the laboratory to the field (e.g. Dasgupta and Stout, 2012), implicit bias (of the type described by Fiske and Molm) is ubiquitous. The challenge for the researcher is to develop the right methodological strategy to capture it and identify its causes. The remedy for subtle/implicit prejudice is usually thought to be 'greater awareness',[6] which

> might make perceivers more mindful of the subtle impact of bias on their judgments and actions and activate corrective processes. At the same time, greater awareness might make targets of discrimination more able to deflect bias by disproving stereotypes when they become aware of it.
> (Dasgupta and Stout, 2012, p. 407)

As I have shown elsewhere (Tileagă, 2005, 2006), and as Roma studies scholarship and activism has also intimated, when it comes to the Roma, *everyone* seems to agree that Roma are unlike any other minority group, and as a consequence warrant 'special' treatment.

It matters less to know whether these prejudices are automatic, or just activated to suit the circumstances. It matters less to locate prejudices and people on a continuum from unconditional tolerance to unqualified intolerance, with a vast middle described by automatic, ambivalent or unconscious prejudices. Prejudices continue to be prejudices – anti-Roma prejudices are prejudices of collective definition; they are prejudices not tied to automatic psychological processes; they are prejudices closely tied to evaluating the moral *worth* of people usually described as Roma/Gypsies.

In natural discourse, everyday conversations, in media reports, newspaper columns, televised debates, etc., Roma stereotypes are used to construct various negative and positive images of individuals, groups and communities, which most often clash with Roma self-representations. The stereotypical image of the Roma in Europe depicts them as failing the various tests of 'worth' that societies impose on their citizens. They are described as unworthy of equal treatment and as failures on the motivational and moral schemes of societies. More worryingly, they are portrayed as a problem without a solution. Ethnologists, anthropologists and ethnographers have shown the power of romantic and folkloric images of Gypsies/Roma (see Okely, 1983) that include both idealization (romanticization) as well as stigmatization (diabolization) (Kligman, 2001). The influence of literature (for example, the British romanticism of Walter Scott and the German romanticism of Nikolaus Lenau) played a major part in the sedimentation of stereotypical romantic images of otherness.

When stereotypical images are pitted against self-descriptions, the problem of self-definition and identification with the Roma in-group (to which I turn in Chapter 4) creates quandaries for people who describe themselves as 'Gypsy'. Here are the words of a Romanian Roma activist Valeriu Nicolae,[7] which capture nicely the tension between stereotypes and self-definition:

> In Europe, when I give this answer, people look at me like I am crazy. Gypsies are the people no one wants around: the thieves and the beggars who cheat everybody and live rich and carefree lives. But I was the manager of a respectable company with partners all over the continent. I did not prominently display any big gold rings or chains; in fact, I seemed to be absolutely normal. In North America the reaction when I say I am a Gypsy is usually 'cool!' They think I must be a free spirit with some mystical ability to read their future in their palms, even though I work as a programmer. None of them know or want to know that life for the majority of Roma in Romania is a daily struggle for survival and nothing else … I didn't see anyone playing music or dancing close to the garbage dump or the canteen garbage bins. There were no tarot card readers or beautiful dramatic girls after the market closed. In the orphanages I found no free and open fields or passionate lifestyles. But there are Gypsies: there are thousands of them just trying to find a way to survive through the day. Some of the kids have enormous, dramatic brown eyes but it is just despair or fever flickering in those eyes.

What Valeriu Nicolae describes is a world where, depending on the social context, stereotypes are the reflection of both negative, old-fashioned and naive, yet well-intentioned, prejudices. Both kinds of prejudices pre-judge 'reality' – they ignore the actual living conditions and the everyday struggles of Gypsies. Valeriu Nicolae writes about an everyday reality that reaches beyond stereotypes – what pains him are prejudices that stem from ignoring the tragic marginality and predicament of Gypsies; prejudices that stem from the ignorance of Gypsies' moral worth. It can be said that discourses that ignore the tragic marginality and everyday predicament of Gypsies are moral discourses. The reverse of prejudices that stem from ignorance are prejudices where the Roma/Gypsies are directly blamed for their predicament. These are prejudices that mingle discourses of social and moral inferiority with wider socio-political discourses around the preservation of rights and freedoms for the majority, the 'settled', the 'civilized'. These are discourses that are steeped in the history and political imaginary of Europe itself, the history of its political ideologies and, more recently, the history and the politics of an enlarged European Union.

In one of the most honest and penetrating analyses of modern European racism, Michel Wieviorka (1995) opens the argument with the question: 'Is it not the case that, at the end of the twentieth century, France is becoming a racist society?' As a sociologist, Wieviorka recognizes that what might lurk under the surface of his (sociological) analysis of racism might be the uneasy realization that racism might be indeed a problem.[8] Wieviorka's hypothesis was that

> the present upsurge in racism, both in France and in other European societies, is not dissociable from a significant social mutation ... modernity is so badly shaken today ... states seem increasingly powerless to maintain the old models of integration; and everywhere communal identities, whether defined in religious, ethnic, regional, cultural, historical, or more importantly, national terms, are emerging or being reinforced.
>
> (Ibid., p. xi)

In a similar fashion one could ask: Is it not the case that European societies are becoming racist societies? In order to even start answering the question one needs, first, to start understanding the new nature of marginality in Europe brought about by the expansion of the European Union.[9] European enlargement, with its promise of freedom of movement, freedom of settlement, has elicited various kinds of discourses and responses from established European democracies and newcomers to the European project. Both before and after the successive waves of accession (in 2004 and 2007), as Stewart notes,

> across Europe polities face: a rising tide of xenophobia; a feeling of loss of sovereignty and democratic oversight; disillusionment with existing political elites ... these all ... promote a wave of anxieties that will, in certain circumstances, be used to turn the Roma into a suitable "target population" to which fears and frustrations can be attached.
>
> (2012a, p. xxxviii)

Because of the uniqueness of historical persecution, prejudices against Roma/Gypsies are vulnerable to the 'resurfacing' of prejudices that reproduce their historical and social marginality.

Roma/Gypsies' historical marginality has gone through different stages, from brutal treatment in medieval times to communism's attempt to state-manage their socio-economic marginality by transforming them into socialist workers.[10] The fall of communism in Europe led to uneven emancipation and empowerment but without significant improvement of their economic and social marginality. As the European Union was becoming stronger and bigger, so were the attempts to fight Roma poverty, destitution, unemployment and lack of opportunities in education and health, and, generally, to encourage affirmative action across the board. But the new, enlarged Europe was not only trying to fight inequalities but, with its new populist and 'integralist' politics and its models of technocratic governance, was also encouraging the creation of new regimes of 'advanced marginality' (Wacquant, 2008), including, but not limited to, residential segregation. In Chapter 6 I show how segregation, especially residential segregation, diminishes and degrades the dignity of Romani people.

A close analysis of marginality can show that racism against Gypsies is not simply a matter of stereotyping and negative evaluation or individual differences, but rather a matter 'rooted in a long legal, administrative and policing tradition' (About, 2012, p. 114), with myriad symbolic connections and ramifications. The critical framework outlined in Chapter 1 offers the means of analysing the special kind of racism to which Roma are subjected; a kind of racism where marginality is the direct, and sometimes indirect, result of social and societal mechanisms of altering and transforming people's worth and dignity.

Notes

1 What Glick calls 'envious prejudice' can be used to 'explain' the occurrence and long history of extreme forms of prejudice and genocide throughout history, but does 'envious prejudice' really explain all manifestations of extreme prejudice?
2 American culture (values, norms, assumptions, habitus) feeds the conflict between the American creed and beliefs and behaviours that oppose positive discrimination and further domination and oppression.
3 According to Nier and Gaertner (2012), the contemporary challenge of detecting contemporary forms of discrimination (race and gender) is to be able to capture and describe its particularly subtle and often unintentional nature.
4 One might argue that Fiske and Molm are not saying anything different from modern racism approaches. They might be using a different vocabulary, but essentially, the message is the same. Yet their claims are bolder and far-reaching. They share the same belief in the power of psychological science in distinguishing between prejudices and people, but Fiske and Molm go a step further by attempting to offer a psychological model that can be used to predict the variety of (everyday) discriminatory behaviour.
5 But see Mitchell and Tetlock (2006) and Tetlock and Mitchell (2009) for persuasive critiques of subtle bias perspectives.
6 One of the problems with this view is that it does not seem to take into account the existing and active awareness of targets of discrimination and does not

square with victims' perceptions and descriptions of racism, and alternative (non-psychological) views about how racism circulates and is circulated in society (see, for instance, Hill, 2008 for an influential account of the linguistic complexity of white racism).

7 http://kopachi.com/archives/articles/authors/valeriu-nicolae.

8 As does Memmi, Wieviorka believes that racism is an action, with 'its representations, its active behaviours, its political expressions, its modes of mobilization, its history … its memory … its inflections and fluctuations' (1995, p. 124), but not one that 'can be studied in itself, without taking other actions into consideration' (ibid.). Racism manifests itself within individual, social or communal (national) configurations of practices.

9 I return to the issue of marginality in Chapter 6 where I discuss the relationship between marginality and moral transgression.

10 For accounts of Roma/Gypsy marginality through history, see Fraser (1992); for Roma/Gypsies under communism, see Barany (2002, ch. 4).

Chapter 3

Personality and racism as predisposition

In the previous chapter I explored some of the most important lines of thought in the social psychology of stereotyping and modern racism. I argued that understanding anti-Roma racism is not simply a matter of considering negative stereotypes as biased attitudinal products or subsuming it under the heading of 'modern'/'new' racism, but rather attending to the presence and nature of Roma marginality as a result of implicit and explicit societal mechanisms of altering, transforming, people's worth and dignity. When discussing modern racist approaches I remarked how the changing nature of racism engenders new human types and typologies. The conventional psychological view of modern racism starts with the idea that, in order to understand racism, one needs to gain a deeper understanding of individual differences between people. The multiple varieties of racism (modern, symbolic, laissez-faire, colour-blind, etc.) map onto categories or types of people that fare differently on indices or measures of tolerance/intolerance.

In this chapter I want to discuss the role of personality in understanding the complexity of prejudice, racism and discrimination in general, and anti-Roma prejudice, racism and discrimination in particular. I start by examining the contribution of the perspective of the 'authoritarian personality' (Adorno *et al.*, 1982 [1950]), and then I move on to more recent developments in personality research by looking at the concept of the 'authoritarian dynamic' (Stenner, 2005) and the contemporary resurgence of the Big Five model (Mondak, 2010) in understanding social and political behaviour. I close the chapter with a discussion of two principal limitations of the personality approach and exegesis: (1) its inability to explain the uniformity of prejudice and racism in society, and their historical specificity; and (2) its failure to explain the variability, existence and ideological force of different types of prejudices.

The most recognizable (and most enduring) psychological human type is Adorno *et al.*'s authoritarian type of person. In Chapter 2 I mentioned the 'authoritarian personality' as an example of stereotyping as a pathology of individual cognition, and as reflecting a general prejudiced attitude with an intra-psychic, psychodynamic source. Here I want to assess its contemporary value, and what we can still learn from it. Are there any aspects that have been overrated or unjustly ignored? How has the 'authoritarian personality' perspective been reinterpreted, completed, by contemporary researchers? How useful is it when applied to understanding real-world, societal manifestations of prejudice, racism and discrimination against the Roma?

Adorno *et al.*'s focus on authoritarianism can be seen as a reaction to a psychological view that presents people as, fundamentally, not different from each other. For instance, Myrdal (1996 [1944], p. 1023) expresses this view aptly:

> behind all outward dissimilarities, behind their contradictory valuations, rationalizations, vested interests, group allegiances and animosities, behind fears and defense constructions, behind the role they play in life and the mask they wear, people are all much alike on a fundamental level. And they are all good people. They want to be rational and just. They all plead to their conscience that they meant well even when things went wrong. Social study is concerned with explaining why all these potentially and intentionally good people so often make life a hell for themselves and each other when they live together, whether in a family, a community, a nation or a world.

In contrast, for Adorno *et al.*, people are not 'potentially and intentionally good people' but rather potentially and intentionally 'bad', corrupted by their inner psychology and impulses, and by strict and conformist rearing practices in highly hierarchized societies. The authoritarian type of person is depicted as the prejudiced, dogmatic person that has to resolve a number of intra-psychic conflicts, and for whom the choice of a particular target group for the projection of aggressive and destructive impulses (tendencies) is secondary. Its counter-type is Allport's 'democratic person'. The democratic person (or 'tolerant personality') is characterized by a 'friendly and trustful attitude' towards others (regardless of group), 'empathic ability', 'self-insight' and 'tolerance for ambiguity' (Allport, 1954).

For Adorno *et al.*, the problem of research on prejudices and discrimination in society revolved around developing and promoting

> an understanding of social-psychological factors which have made it possible for the authoritarian type of man to threaten to replace the individualistic and democratic type prevalent in the past century and a half of our civilization, and of the factors by which this threat may be contained.
> (1982 [1950], p. x)

Although still interested in human types, Allport presented a more nuanced picture. For him, prejudiced, as well as tolerant, individuals belonged to different types. For instance, Allport identifies several human types that go along with different types of prejudice and tolerance. Conformists, 'swayed' by the tolerant or prejudiced group norm, take the path of either *conformity* prejudice or tolerance, whereas those with a positive or negative 'state of personality organization' would adopt *character-conditioned* prejudice or tolerance.[1]

Both Adorno *et al.* and Allport believed in the power of interiority, of inner life and organization of 'personality'. Both believed that one could not understand the nature of prejudices if one could not design/construct a way to tell people apart, to pigeonhole them based on a definite set of psychological characteristics. For both Adorno *et al.* and Allport, prejudiced, as well as tolerant, thinking reflected the *total* style of 'personality' organization and operation, a 'reflection of a total style of cognitive operation' (Allport, 1954, p. 438).

But how easy it is to distinguish, for instance, between conformity prejudice or tolerance and character-conditioned prejudice or tolerance? How easy is it to keep human types apart when analysing real-world manifestations of racism? How are we to describe and explain the explicit or implicit ambivalence of authoritarians, or the subtle prejudice of the tolerant personality?

Adorno *et al.* and Allport have introduced an individual differences approach to understanding prejudices in society through a focus on the inner world of the individual. When life is full of painful threats, and a conscious strong self does not negotiate these threats satisfactorily, psychological insecurity and inner conflicts take hold of an individual, and the seed of an authoritarian personality is planted. In contrast, a democratic and 'mature' personality is 'largely a matter of building inner security' (Allport, 1954, p. 441).

Starting from the rather simple question of why competing political ideologies have such differing degrees of appeal for different individuals (see Adorno *et al.*, 1950, p. 2), Adorno *et al.* were interested in charting individual differences in ideological affiliation. Adorno *et al.*'s basic hypothesis was that the political and social attitudes of an individual cluster together and are the expression of 'deep lying trends in personality' (ibid., p. 1). The assumption behind Adorno *et al.*'s analysis was that 'prejudiced people are those whose personalities render them susceptible to those racist or fascist ideas prevalent in a society at a given time' (Brown, 1995, p. 19). They were interested to describe the authoritarian personality of the potential fascist with an emphasis on the role of psychodynamic and cognitive factors on the construction and expression of social attitudes. The 'authoritarian personality' was described as a complex syndrome of behaviours, attitudes and dispositions, characterized by an over-rigid cognitive style, which does not easily accommodate ambivalence and ambiguity, conventionalism, authoritarian submission and aggression, stereotypy and destructiveness.

Adorno *et al.* also emphasized the role of conformist and highly hierarchized society in the crystallization of a general psychological orientation (syndrome of intolerance).[2] There is compatibility between a conformist, highly hierarchized culture and the nature of individual psychology it creates.

Close scrutiny of Adorno *et al.*'s theoretical and methodological presuppositions has revealed a range of methodological and theoretical flaws (Brown, 1965; Christie and Jahoda, 1954; Rokeach, 1956; see also Altemeyer, 1981; Billig, 1978). Problems were identified with the design and validation of the F-scale and reported correlations with variables such as intelligence, social class or level of education, which suggest alternative explanations for the genesis of authoritarianism. For example, Altemeyer (1981) argues that the nine components said to comprise authoritarianism are too vague and he offers evidence in support of the idea that successive factor-analytic studies have failed to uncover the nine dimensions that are said to form the core of 'authoritarianism'.[3]

Adorno *et al.*'s general claim was that it is possible to measure prejudice by describing the 'authoritarian' personality without reference to any specific ethnic group. Yet, research by Diab (1959) has demonstrated that authoritarianism may predict prejudice towards some groups but not others. In his study, authoritarianism predicted prejudice towards Jews, but not towards other groups. Research conducted by Pettigrew (1958) in South Africa and the Southern United States has offered evidence that in some cultures the pressure to conform to racist views is so powerful that it has a significant effect on personal beliefs. In cultures where prejudiced attitudes are generally tolerated and where (prejudiced) group norms hold strong sway, even if not endorsed by all, personality characteristics have a much less prominent influence on the creation and the perpetuation of prejudiced attitudes. Situational norms, intergroup contact and relations with others were proved to have a more critical influence than personality dispositions (e.g. Minard, 1952; Siegel and Siegel, 1957).

The influence of situational and group norms, as well as the salience of social identities (Reynolds and Turner, 2001; see also Haslam and Wilson, 2000; Verkuyten and Hagendoorn, 1998), can describe, with much more accuracy, the various complex social manifestations of prejudice. Explaining prejudice in the way that Adorno *et al.* intended – through individual differences between people – fails to capture not only why, but how prejudices reproduce themselves at broader cultural, societal and historical levels, and may persist as ruling collective ideology in certain societies.

Researchers have also argued that authoritarianism does not operate as a separate dimension. Intolerance is the product of a cluster of 'social attitudinal expressions' that include authoritarianism, conservatism and traditionalism (Duckitt *et al.*, 2010). As an attitudinal dimension, authoritarianism is operationalized as belief in coercive social control, but different social contexts (especially those that have undergone rapid and traumatic social change) may present different patterns. Also, as Duckitt *et al.* (2010) argued, when one considers different types of authoritarians one notices substantial differences in traditionalism and conservatism.

Dynamic authoritarianism and threat

More recent approaches consider authoritarianism as a psychological dimension that is 'activated' or 'deactivated' by different conditions, circumstances and social contexts. Allport's early (although not exclusive) concern with a certain 'type of "character-structure" that resorts to prejudice when threats are felt' (1950, p. 12) was taken forward by researchers who considered intolerance as an effect of the dynamic interaction between personality, environment and threat. A wealth of research has shown how dislike of, antipathy towards, social groups is mediated by realistic and symbolic threats and intergroup anxiety (Stephan *et al.*, 1998, 2000, 2002). Duckitt *et al.* (2010, p. 708) have demonstrated how authoritarianism, conservatism and traditionalism were associated with different kinds social threat. As they argued, authoritarianism was more likely to predict concerns about 'direct physical threats to social and personal safety, well being and security', conservatism was more likely to predict 'concerns about threats to social cohesion, harmony, and consensus', whereas traditionalism predicted 'concerns about the threat of social changes that disrupt and undermine traditional lifestyles and morality'. Other researchers went a step further and argued that changing conditions of threat, interacting with a deep-seated predisposition towards authoritarianism, provide a better explanatory leverage for understanding intolerance across ethnic and national groups, and across socio-political contexts (Stenner, 2005). As Stenner argues, manifestations of authoritarianism 'depend upon the *interaction* of individual predispositions with threatening societal conditions' (ibid., p. 26, italics in original). At the core of Stenner's authoritarian dynamic lies a belief in individual differences and proclivity for intolerance of difference. Stenner contends that 'individuals posses fairly stable predispositions to intolerance of difference, that is, varying levels of willingness to "put up with" differing people, ideas, and behaviors' (ibid., p. 2). Moreover, the authoritarian predisposition 'seems to be a relatively innate and enduring individual trait' (ibid., p. 326).

According to Stenner, differences of style of thinking can differentiate between people who can be categorized as 'libertarians' or 'authoritarians'. 'Authoritarians' and 'libertarians' can also be differentiated in terms of their 'cognitive capacity' when discussing social issues such as racism, religion, etc. In Stenner's words, 'in these "natural" conversations, the libertarians proved to be a good deal more cognitively complex that authoritarians under any conditions' (2005, p. 234). Different cognitive styles reflect 'innate capacities of the individuals' (ibid., p. 235). Interestingly, Stenner does not seem to be concerned with whatever might be found in the middle of a continuum between 'libertarians' and 'authoritarians' – the 'vast middle' that Fiske and Molm (2010) are writing about. Instead, she is more concerned with the social and political conditions (peculiar to American democracy) – 'amplification of conflict', the 'propagation of adversaries' and 'the constant airing of disagreement' – whose role is to 'activate' the authoritarian dynamic.

She is more concerned with how democracy can be made 'more secure' and tolerance 'maximized' by designing 'systems to accommodate how people actually are. Because some people will never live comfortably in a modern liberal democracy' (Stenner, 2005, p. 335). But, as I will be arguing in this chapter, a belief in a putative essence that resides in people, a narrow focus on 'how people actually are', does not advance much the discussion around the tragic, societal dilemma of racism. Liberal democracy does not just facilitate the expression of intolerant attitudes steeped in authoritarian predispositions, as Stenner would have it, but is the cradle for innumerable societal arrangements that mediate and influence how we treat and judge the worth of others, regardless of putative inner predispositions.

Personality, psychological predispositions and traits

A different perspective on individual differences is offered by what some psychologists call a 'broadscale trait approach' (Mondak, 2010), and the role of psychological predispositions in social and political behaviour. This is a move beyond authoritarianism to a more holistic approach to personality as 'consequential at multiple levels and in multiple ways' (ibid., p. 146), and defined as 'a stable, biologically influenced psychological structure' (ibid., p. 183). The focus is on personality traits (openness to experience, conscientiousness, extraversion, agreeableness and emotional stability – the 'Big Five') that are seen to play an important role in the acquisition of political information, political participation and regulation of political predispositions. The Big Five approach takes seriously not only the interaction between personality and environmental factors, but also the role of 'innate biological or biologically influenced factors, and interactions between environmental and innate forces' (ibid., p. 182). Personality (its various dimensions) is the axis around which the impact of biology and social conditions on ideology operates. Direct, positive relationships are found between political attitudes and personality traits such as openness to experience, conscientiousness and agreeableness. Across a range of American national surveys, greater 'openness to experience' is seen to correlate with ideological liberalism, whereas 'conscientiousness' is seen to correlate with conservatism. Extraversion and agreeableness have no noteworthy impact on political ideology. Yet, extraversion produces a noticeable impact on a variety of forms of political participation, with openness to experience also playing a worthwhile role. The Big Five do seem to have direct effects on prejudice. Sibley and Duckitt (2008) argue that effects of 'agreeableness' on prejudice are mediated by social dominance orientation, whereas the effects of 'openness to experience' are, to a large extent, mediated by right-wing authoritarianism.

Whereas for Stenner the relative influence of threat and personality leads to the identification of definite human (psychological) types ('libertarians' and 'authoritarians'), for Mondak, it is the relative ratio/combination of (five) personality traits that describes 'emerging' psychological types: the 'conservative' and the 'liberal'. As Mondak argues, 'the conservative is an individual who is conscientious, level-headed, and fixed in his or her ways', whereas the 'the liberal exhibits less psychological reliability and stability than the conservative, but has a greater tendency to embrace new ideas, and perhaps a slight proclivity to be relatively warm and agreeable' (2010, p. 130).

For both Stenner and Mondak it is people's psychobiological 'nature' that predisposes them to be 'libertarians'/'liberals' or 'authoritarians'/'co nservatives'. Both are more interested in the extremes of the continuum tolerance/intolerance than in the 'vast middle'. Yet, as I will be arguing in the remainder of this chapter, tolerant as well as intolerant attitudes are not simply the outcome of psychobiological predispositions (whether or not in interaction with threat or the environment). Any understanding of the societal dilemmas of racism in general, as well as its particularistic manifestations in the case of the Roma, requires a move away from categorizing people in terms of tolerant or intolerant predispositions. Moving away from the extremes of the spectrum implies finding novel ways of approaching the analysis of the 'vast middle', the grey areas of subtle prejudice, that take into account the role of collective assumptions about society, the meaning of prejudice, nationhood and other societal aspects that influence how we treat and judge the worth of others.

Extreme prejudice as collective definition

Psychological research on authoritarianism has opened the way for analyses of a variety of intensities of prejudices that are not so much contingent on the nature of the object of prejudice as upon individual pathology, an individual's socialization experiences and beliefs about authority and dominance in society, psychodynamic factors, psychological motivations and needs. For instance, a wealth of research studies in the 'hate crimes' literature provides evidence that 'perpetrators of hate crimes have distinctive views about authority, and in some cases, may experience psychopathology as a result of early socialization experiences' (Craig, 2002, p. 97). Although the majority of individuals studied are not members of organized hate groups, deep-seated resentment, disgust, envy, frustration and continuous anti-minority sentiment are part of the clinical tableau.[4]

When one turns to public discourse about Roma in the public sphere, one can identify many instances of extreme anti-minority views. The online English edition of the German newspaper *Spiegel* reported recently a commentary by prominent Hungarian conservative public figure, and founder of Hungary's ruling party, Zsolt Bayer, following a bar brawl in a small town near Budapest when two young Hungarian athletes were seriously wounded by a group of Roma:

> A significant part of the Roma are unfit for coexistence. They are not fit to live among people. These Roma are animals, and they behave like animals. When they meet with resistance, they commit murder. They are incapable of human communication. Inarticulate sounds pour out of their bestial skulls. At the same time, these Gypsies understand how to exploit the 'achievements' of the idiotic Western world. But one must retaliate rather than tolerate. These animals shouldn't be allowed to exist. In no way. That needs to be solved – immediately and regardless of the method.
>
> (Verseck, 2013)

Both the layperson and social psychologist would be inclined to ask the same question: What *kind* of person is Bayer? What *drives* him to say those horrible things about Roma? Is Bayer the kind of prejudiced person for whom it matters less which group prejudice is directed against? This chapter has singled out one type of answer to these questions: an answer that emphasizes the role of individual differences and individual pathology. In the next sections (and subsequent chapters) I propose an alternative view that reframes these very questions and potential answers to them. How far can the notion of intolerance derived from personality or 'relatively intransient psychological orientations' (Mondak, 2010, p. 21) take us in understanding extreme prejudice against Roma? How important is it to understand what kind of person or what human type Bayer belongs to?

One might be tempted to say, following personality theorists, that the Hungarian commentator exhibits some enduring tendencies, or traits, that are a 'poor fit' for a tolerant attitude. He could be described as belonging to the type of rigid, psychologically insecure, close-minded ideologue, dogmatic, unreflective authoritarian. As noted earlier, personality theorists agree that by 'knowing something about a person's general psychological tendencies, we potentially would be able to enrich our understanding of … [a] person's specific behaviors and attitudes' (Mondak, 2010, p. 1). If we were to follow this route we would be able to infer Bayer's conservative politics from psychologically rooted predispositions.

Other psychologists might describe Bayer as the 'ill-intentioned extremist', at the opposite end of the continuum from the 'well-intentioned moderate'

(Fiske, 2002). Bayer expresses 'blatant biases' that are 'conscious, hot, direct, and unambiguous'. Moreover, he could be described as an 'extremist' because he perceives the Roma as a threat to the in-group's life and values (Stephan *et al.*, 2008), and, implicitly, espouses the view that superior groups should dominate inferior groups (Sidanius and Pratto, 1999).

A perhaps more profitable alternative would be to move away from speculating about Bayer's personality and consider closely the tone and organization of his discourse. When focusing on personality we tend to separate the 'individual' from the 'social actor'. Although it is usually argued that only subtle prejudices are complex, whereas blatant prejudices are hot-blooded, direct and unambiguous, I also want to argue here that we should not discount too hastily the inherent complexity of extreme or blatant prejudices (Billig, 1978; Tileagă, 2013). The meaning of extremism varies across individuals and social contexts (cf., inter alia, Hopkins and Kahani-Hopkins, 2009; Ferguson *et al.*, 2008; Klandermans and Mayer, 2006). Also, researchers have shown that right-wing attitudes do not show a strong correlation with psychological ill-being, and are less likely to stem from personal anxieties (Onraet and van Hiel, 2014).

The ill-intentioned extremist belongs to every society's collection of social/human types – it is not a universal psychological type. The ill-intentioned extremist (like the well-intentioned moderate) is, first and foremost, a social actor who is not a passive recipient of ideology (Billig *et al.*, 1988). He is a social agent who engages with the prevailing ideology of the times. Intolerance is more a matter of collective definition than of personality (Tileagă, 2014). Bayer finds reasons with a basis in collective assumptions about the acceptability and reasonableness of extreme prejudices against the Roma, rather than his own subjectivity (Tileagă, 2005).

Bayer does not simply adopt an opinion (that may or may not be in keeping with his personality), he 'chooses himself as a person' (Sartre, 1995 [1948], p. 53). Although we may be able to sketch a personality profile for Bayer, we may miss the crux of his rhetoric. If we simply assumed that the language he uses is in keeping with his 'personality' or 'character', then we would miss a lot of consequential detail regarding the tone and organization of his speech.

His tone is not of irritated distance but a tone of action. Bayer is the man of action that demands urgent and decisive action against the Roma. He tries to appeal to the sensibilities of his compatriots, to those who feel dispossessed or let down by the European project. Bayer's diatribe mingles extreme anti-Roma sentiment with anti-Europeanism. One does not talk about the Roma in a vacuum, but there is always a context (local, national, cross-national), the backdrop against which the Roma are said to be worthy or, like in this case, unworthy of coexistence. The point of his rhetoric is to make a case for reasonable discrimination. Hostile discourse and actions need a framework of reasonableness.

Bayer's words reproduce a cultural conception of racism that crosses national borders. Bayer is not talking about Hungary in particular, and Hungary's Roma, but he issues a collective call to action that concerns the collective *social category* Roma. The Roma are not simply an adversary group like in the case of intractable conflicts (cf. Bar-Tal and Teichman, 2005), but a group (described as) unlike any other. Their description does not fit the typical psychological (intergroup) repertoire of group animosity or antipathy that characterizes anti-immigrant discourse or envious prejudice. Bayer is not merely making a factual observation about the Roma; he offers a (collective) *justification* for why Roma ought to be treated differently and relegated to a subhuman condition.

The eliminationist conclusion ('these animals shouldn't be allowed to exist. In no way. That needs to be solved – immediately and regardless of the method') connects Bayer to a (national and global) history of Roma persecution. He contends that anyone in possession of the clear 'facts' about the Roma would come to the same conclusion. To focus on presumably flawed or irrational psychology would mean to miss the crux and the ideological implications of such claims.

Extreme views such as Bayer's do not reflect a psychological dimension of 'authoritarianism'; they reflect a deeper historical mentality and stance towards the Roma – historical group persecution. Drawing on Ruth Benedict, Moscovici (2011) contends that persecution is a much older story, in place long before the current modern vocabulary of racism and anti-racism. Paradoxically, thus, we don't need to investigate racism, but what comes before it – the history of persecution from which it originates. Persecution is a historical, anthropological and ethnographic issue, whereas racism is primordially considered a psychological issue. Even a cursory inspection of the historical record of Roma persecution in Europe can reveal the reasons why Bayer's words are so dangerous. And those reasons have nothing to do with his or someone else's personality.

Discourses such as Bayer's can be multiplied at will. They crop up on message boards, in blogs, in news interviews, at political meetings and in political speeches, around the dinner table, all around Europe. Bayer's words are not a one-off expression of discontent or frustration with the Roma. These discourses are the discourses of a culture where a society's common-sense 'stock' of prejudices, experiences and knowledge about worth and dignity are used to operate distinctions between those who are worthy to be treated as human beings and those who are not. In Europe, more often than not, these are discourses of the 'vast middle', of people who are usually thought of as trading in subtle, ambiguous and ambivalent prejudices, rather than 'hot-minded' or 'bloody-minded' prejudices. It is comfortable to think of the prejudices of the 'middle' as subtle rather than extreme, to think of them as automatic, implicit and/or unconscious rather than as cultural prejudices. It is vital that we understand not only the subtle prejudices, but also the extreme prejudices of the 'vast middle', which are, of course, not without their ambiguities or contradictions.

People like Bayer will air very different prejudices when talking about groups other than the Roma. For instance, conventional anti-immigrant prejudices, and anti-immigration 'bias', documented by various researchers, is strikingly different from the extreme prejudices against the Roma. Whereas anti-immigrant bias is explained in terms of intergroup competition for material resources and identities, threat, negative emotions and dynamics of national identification (for a review, see Wagner *et al.*, 2013), extreme prejudices against the Roma present strikingly peculiar eliminationist and dehumanizing contours.

When Europeans like Bayer are talking about the Roma they can freely reproduce a societal consensus that says Roma are unfit for coexistence, subhuman, failures according to the many motivational and moral schemes of society, not worthy of equal and democratic treatment. Europeans like Bayer reproduce a societal consensus that says that it is acceptable to be unapologetically racist when it comes to the Roma. This societal consensus has roots in a specific history of persecution and anthropological repertoires of European societies (Fraser, 1992).

The Roma are the archetypal 'problem-group' that suffers from the historical curse of persecution (Stewart, 2012a). Persecution is tightly linked to authority – the authority to instigate, control and sanction actions that solve the problems related to the (unwanted) presence of others. The macro-context of historical persecution provides a useful vantage point for understanding the resurgence of authority calls that demand undemocratic solutions to social problems posed by the presence of unworthy others.

From psychological differences to the societal repertories of liberal democratic societies

Personality researchers contend that

> different points of view survive, and even thrive ... in no small part because people are not all the same ... the reason people are not all on the same political page is ... because people exhibit fundamental and persistent psychological differences, differences that are largely rooted in biology.
>
> (Mondak, 2010, p. 131)

The notion of 'persistent psychological differences' is a key explanatory principle with a long and venerable history in social psychology. But what persistent psychological differences cannot satisfactorily explain is the historical and cultural specificity of certain social and political points of view.

Another limitation of any personality account is its inability to explain the uniformity of prejudiced attitudes across the political spectrum, and how prejudices and racism can be sustained and can survive as consensual social representations in certain societies. Personality theory neglects the role of socio-structural factors in the etiology of prejudice. It also 'pathologizes both the ideology and the characters who endorse it, thus severely limiting the range of critical investigation' (Wetherell and Potter, 1992, p. 56).

More importantly, understanding the argumentative nature of holding strong or extreme points of view cannot be simply explained with reference to psychological differences. Racist and exclusionary legitimations of the status quo do not always work through the inflexibility of the authoritarian mode of thinking. In Chapters 5, 6 and 7 I will be showing how discourse analyses can reveal the inherent complexity, and flexibility, of racist legitimations of social formations and unequal power relations. In Chapter 4 I will be arguing that prejudiced personalities are not given, once and for all, 'formed and fixed in the past but can reflect contemporary group activities and associated processes of social influence' (Reynolds and Turner, 2006, p. 263). As cross-situational effects of psychological differences are mixed, and sometimes inconclusive, it is difficult not to take into account situated contexts of identity and racism as a discursive product. If, as Bandura writes, 'the massive threats to human welfare stem mainly from deliberate acts of principle rather than from unrestrained acts of impulse' (1999, p. 207), then one may need to rethink the presumed primacy of traits or psychological predispositions over values (Caprara *et al.*, 2006), social identities (Reynolds and Turner, 2006) or discourse (Tileagă, 2005, 2013).

Extreme views that we tend to attribute to personality are, arguably, part and parcel of reasoned collective argument(s). In the rhetoric of extreme prejudice, argument and thinking are intimately tied. Thinking refers to a process of collective thinking. As discursive psychologists have shown, public rhetoric is the 'driver' of collective definitions of social issues and social problems (Tileagă, 2014). The categories of extreme ideologies of the (seemingly decent) 'vast middle' are framed in the societal and historical repertories around worth, dignity and moral exclusion of liberal democratic societies.

If extremism is both a 'passion and a conception of the world' (Sartre, 1995 [1948], p. 17), then what is the source of people's conception of the world? Societal and historical repertoires of liberal democracies feed 'extreme' conceptions of the world (including the meaning of 'extremism'). These conceptions are not individual; they are collective, imparted and shared with others (Jovchelovitch, 2007).

It would be far-fetched to argue that the extreme prejudices of the 'vast middle' are the result of some deep-seated predisposition to hate; rather they are social products of liberal democracies. Extreme views such as the ones presented in this chapter are easily recognizable as anti-democratic feelings, because what is at stake is not negative stereotyping nor listing negative attributes of the Roma, but demanding undemocratic, eliminationist solutions for a 'problem group'. They also exhibit a sense of moral superiority and self-righteousness. The problem of some of today's European societies is that extreme prejudice and moral exclusion thrives in liberal democracies, within the framework (and protection) offered by the nation-state.

In their search for 'representative' psychological types psychologists tend to overestimate the internal consistency of ideologies of prejudice. As the next chapters will show, the language that people use, the rhetorical choices they make, the emphasis placed on some aspects of ideology rather than others, the social identity positions they inhabit, uncover a more complex psychological reality that goes beyond the psychological properties of individuals. If we simply dismiss the Hungarian commentator as an 'ill-intentioned extremist' or relegate him to a specific personality type, we restrict the kinds of critical questions that we can ask about the creation and reproduction of extreme prejudice against and moral exclusion of Roma. If we discount the possibility that extreme, morally exclusionary views levelled at the Roma may be expressed by people across the political spectrum, and not just by 'extremists', then we will fail to understand why, and how, extreme prejudices against the Roma persist.

The ideology of extreme prejudice belongs to the category of 'performative' rather than 'constative' language (Eagleton, 1991, p. 19). As a consequence, it is more helpful to view the ideology of extreme prejudice as a 'particular set of *effects* within discourses' (ibid., p. 194, my emphasis). Moral exclusion is one of these pernicious effects. Tileagă (2005, 2006, 2007) identifies a 'consensus' around a moral exclusionary discourse against the Roma in Europe (a discourse that is different from prejudiced discourse about other minorities) that denies the Roma a moral standing in the world, places them outside the boundary where moral values and considerations of humanity, fair treatment and equality apply, and portrays them as expendable. Both participants 'supporting' extremist politics and those 'opposing' it describe the Roma as transgressing civilized conduct and moral conventions, as abject, as repulsive (or inviting repulsion). They are presented as transgressing moral (and spatial) boundaries, and as a consequence are typically classified as matter 'out of place'. For some people, they are the 'scum of society'; for others they are not only 'dirty', they are literally 'dirt'. Various metaphors of residue (dirt, scum, etc.) are used as metaphors for residual people. To categorize Roma as residual, as abject, means ignoring their visible human qualities and invites a conclusion with eliminationist connotations.

As I noted earlier, the words uttered by the Hungarian commentator resonate in each and every country of the European continent. In that sense, they don't pertain to an individual, but to a collective tradition of speaking about the Roma. The commentator's argument is one of collective definition (Blumer, 1971) – that is, it draws upon, and constitutes at the same time, a societal discourse that 'defines' one of its minorities as a *social problem*. As Sartre noted when discussing anti-Semitism, one makes oneself an anti-Semite 'because that is something one cannot be alone' (1995 [1948], p. 22). Similarly, one cannot be anti-Roma alone – one needs to attach oneself to a collective tradition that portrays the Roma as a social problem without a solution.

Tolerance and intolerance are not just the property of the open-minded opposed to the closed-minded person, but are also the upshot of argumentative positions that span the entire political and ideological spectrum of societies. One needs to understand the variety of both intolerant and tolerant discourses that embody the paradoxes of liberal democratic societies. One needs to learn more about which social and cultural resources to mobilize against the normalization of intolerance, what works and what does not. One can achieve this by pointing both to the collective construction and definition of tolerance and intolerance, and to its collective discursive history.

As Allport has suggested, we should not just trust, or follow, our own sense of moral outrage, but 'consult the ethos of a culture' (1954, p. 11), and consider the 'moral evaluation placed by a culture on some of its practices' (ibid., p. 11). But he considered this to be only secondary to what he believed to be primary: the functional and relative independence of prejudice as 'negative, overgeneralized judgment'. He believed that we would be able to describe the variety and intensity of prejudiced attitudes by exploring their psychological function for the structuration of personality. He described prejudiced attitudes as a 'psychological crutch for persons crippled in their encounters with life' (ibid., p. 12). We know now that they can serve group (Tajfel, 1981b) and system-justificatory functions (Jost *et al.*, 2004) as well. It is these latter functions that have more far-reaching implications for understanding the social and societal nature of prejudices in society.

Social psychologists should refocus their theories and methods on exploring the forms and mechanisms of moral evaluation placed by various cultures on some of their practices, especially when those practices ensure the moral exclusion of a certain group of people. The notions of authoritarian and democratic personality, the 'open' and 'closed' mind, are notions that map only the extremes of a social continuum of beliefs. It is the struggle for describing the various psychological characteristics of the 'vast middle' that characterizes much of the contemporary social psychology of racism. In researching the ' vast middle', but not restricting it to psychological correlates, the social psychology of racism can construct a better appreciation of societal underpinnings and consequences of racism. By considering closely the nature of anti-Roma prejudices, especially those of the 'vast middle', social psychologists can extend and broaden their approaches to understanding prejudices of collective definition.

Notes

1 Allport also writes about 'militant' and 'pacifist' tolerance. He describes the tolerant person as 'very likely to be liberal in his [*sic*] political views' (Allport, 1954, p. 431), whereas prejudiced individuals 'are more often conservatives' (ibid.). A 'liberal' is a 'person ... who wants progressive social change ... and tends to take a somewhat optimistic view of human nature – that it can be changed for the better' (ibid.).

2 A variant of Adorno's syndrome of intolerance was labelled the 'closed mind' by Rokeach (1960). Rokeach contrasted the closed mind with the 'open mind' or the psychological stance of the non-prejudiced person.

3 Another criticism of Adorno *et al.* was that they dealt with only one variant of authoritarianism, namely right-wing authoritarianism. The argument that people with other political views are also authoritarian and hence also prejudiced was developed and turned into a systematic psychological theory by Rokeach (1956, 1960).

4 Popular (lay) analyses of racism tend to explain it with reference to individual pathology or psychological or moral 'defect'. As Pettigrew (1996) argues, popular analyses of racism tend to approach societal issues (like the pervasiveness and complexity of prejudice) as if they were 'simply a problem of disturbed individuals' (p. 109). Popular analysis also recognizes that words can hurt or wound, in the same way as some researchers do (Graumann, 1998). Popular analysis of racism embraces wholeheartedly a lay version of individual differences between people and more readily embraces explanations based on individual pathology than those based on socio-structural factors.

Chapter 4

Social categorization and contexts of social identity

Social cognition, individual differences and prejudice

In Chapter 2 I only briefly touched upon the various implications of conceiving stereotypes as the upshot of natural information processing and categorical thinking. In this chapter I want to move the discussion from individual differences and irrational categorizations to natural and discursive processes of social categorization. I start by discussing the role of categorical thinking and cognitive factors in prejudice, implicit attitudes and contemporary extensions and critiques of social identity and self-categorization theories. I then explore the usefulness and consequences of ethnographic studies of identity for understanding issues of Romani self-definition and self-affirmation.

This chapter is not intended as an exhaustive review of the literature, but rather as a foundation for a broader discussion about the nature of contemporary anti-Roma prejudices in Europe.

In Chapter 3 I argued that an individual-differences approach to researching prejudice contends that it is the task of psychological theorizing and measurement to be able to identify and describe different kinds of people holding different kinds of belief. Primarily, one should be able to distinguish between those whose psychological profile does not square with the democratic desiderata of society, and those whose psychological profile is ready to accommodate and internalize society's progressive values. The 'conservative' and the 'liberal', the 'ill-intentioned extremist' and the 'well-intentioned democrat' are well-known human types that populate our social and political environment. Each can be described via either a personality profile or a particular propensity to process social information. Distinguishing between different types of people, with different 'personalities' (as well as different types of prejudices), is an extremely valuable enterprise, yet it paints a social world populated by human types at opposing ends from each other, with a vast grey area in the middle.

Social cognition researchers are more interested in the grey area in the middle; they are interested in the explicit or implicit, conscious or unconscious, deliberate or automatic processing of the individual 'perceiver', the 'average' individual. Although rudiments of an individual-differences ethos can be found in social cognition approaches, these are fundamentally concerned with natural cognitive functioning. Adorno *et al.*'s (1982 [1950]) image of the person corrupted by its personality is turned by social cognition into the image of the rational person biased by individual modalities of processing information (Fiske and Taylor, 1991).[1]

What social psychologists call 'bias' creeps into social life and moderates the relationships we establish with others, the way we perceive and act in the context of intergroup relations.[2] Social psychologists have described bias as universal (Allport, 1954), as well as context-dependent (e.g. Hagendoorn *et al.*, 2001). In psychological terms, bias can be deliberate (explicit) or relatively automatic (implicit), and can take a variety of conventional (Tajfel and Wilkes, 1963) and ambivalent/paternalistic forms (Jackman, 2005; Wagner *et al.*, 2013).

From earlier studies on automatic stereotype activation (Devine, 1989) to standardized measures of implicit prejudice (Greenwald and Banaji, 1995; Banaji and Greenwald, 2013) came the realization that people are not immune to prejudice. 'Good', 'well-intentioned' people have their own 'blind spots', biases they carry within them, given to them by social experience. Social judgements are shaped unconsciously and unintentionally by hidden biases.

Implicit attitudes

In his review of implicit prejudice research, Durrheim (2012) argues that 'the study of implicit cognition ... has shown how deeply meaningful race, gender, and other social category information is to people, and how little prompting it takes for people to think in stereotypical ways' (pp. 181–182). Although strong social norms against the expression of overt prejudice have led to a decline of explicit prejudice in liberal democratic societies, what researchers of implicit prejudice are saying is that prejudice is still 'prevalent in the unconscious mind, ever ready to be activated and used in subtle ways' (ibid., p. 182). Implicit attitudes are 'traces of past experience' (Greenwald and Banaji, 1995, p. 268) in memory. Whereas explicit attitudes are seen as stemming from prejudice operating in conscious 'mode', implicit prejudiced attitudes operate 'unconsciously or automatically, outside the ambit of individual awareness, will or intention, and they are consequently not necessarily motivated by (consciously experienced) negative affect or hostility' (Durrheim, 2012, p. 182).

Standardized implicit measures of bias (such as the well-known Implicit Association Test (IAT)) are considered better tests of bias as they are non-reactive. Yet, implicit bias is measured in reaction times, in response to a task, and not by 'what people do, or by what people say' (Arkes and Tetlock, 2004, p. 275) in particular social contexts. Prejudice is subtly stripped of its contextual significance and relevance, of its material and symbolic underpinnings and consequences. From a psychological point of view there is a certain inevitability associated with the notion of implicit attitudes: *anyone* is accountably, potentially 'prejudiced', because, arguably, *anyone* is bound to 'fail' an implicit association test. If anyone is bound to fail the implicit association test, then the 'test' is no longer a *test*, but rather an instrument of subtle confirmatory analysis.

Although the social psychology of implicit prejudiced attitudes is seen as marking a 'radical break' away from the Allportian negative evaluation ethos, it nonetheless keeps intact one other major presupposition of Allport's social psychology of prejudice: its foundational *psychological* character. Uncovering implicit associations between concepts and schemas in memory entails researching *psychological* prejudice, that is, prejudice that has a firm, universal, psychological basis. The question that has not received a satisfactory answer is how one goes from psychological prejudice to *social* prejudice (actual words, actions, behaviours, feelings towards disadvantaged groups or other social categories such as gender, class, nationality, religion), and understands the complexity of its social and political influence (Drury, 2012).

Allport was aware that prejudice was also more than negative evaluation, and he did not reduce prejudice to a set of innocuous, spontaneous behaviours (e.g. eye gaze duration or non-verbal behaviour in general), but was looking for a more comprehensive framework that, whilst retaining psychological insight at its core, would nonetheless be able to describe and explain a much wider range of real-world situations and behaviours.

There is also an unexplored tension at the heart of the argument that implicit prejudice is functionally independent of actual endorsement of prejudiced attitudes. How can one talk about 'prejudice' or 'discrimination' (as evaluative and interpretive notions) without prejudiced attitudes? In conventional terms, it is attitudes that lead to discrimination. How can someone be prejudiced without endorsing a prejudicial attitude? As some authors have argued, it may be the case that the implicit association test is measuring something other than prejudice (Arkes and Tetlock, 2004). Implicit measures reduce prejudice to a set of non-verbal behavioural outcomes (e.g. Dovidio *et al.*, 2002a). Also, a focus on implicit attitudes does not take into consideration the *manner* in which people are prejudiced, and the social *nature* of those prejudices. For instance, one of the findings of IAT research is that African Americans themselves manifest anti-black prejudice. This is not surprising given that we expect that each group will have not only out-group but also in-group prejudices; that is, negative or derogatory beliefs or feelings about members of their own group. Implicit measures confirm what we already know about social expressions of prejudice – that they can be directed towards out-groups as well as in-groups. Arguably, in order to understand why African Americans may manifest anti-black prejudice one needs to consider more than reaction times.

As Durrheim argues, unresolved tensions at the heart of the implicit prejudice problematic may make the concept lose its political and practical 'edge'. In this context, actual perpetrators of prejudiced and discriminatory behaviours can be excused for doing something that, supposedly, lies beyond their conscious control (see also Billig, 2002a). One of the questions that the social psychology of implicit attitudes raises is who is, then, the 'subject' of prejudice? Is the subject of prejudice merely a cultural dupe, unthinkingly absorbing societal experiences? Or is he/she a social actor, an agent in interaction with others? It is important not to abandon the notion of implicit prejudice as a significant dimension of social behaviour. Instead, it is vital to turn it from a purely cognitive and perceptual notion into a notion researched more in social settings such as social interactions between people. Implicit prejudice needs to be researched less as a *private* outcome of cognitive, categorical associations in memory, and more as a *publicly* accountable outcome of social interactions between people.

The social contexts in which people express their prejudiced evaluations have to be part of the analysis. Instead of being universalized, the prejudiced subject needs to be recognized as a 'fully social subject who can expect to justify their attitudes or behaviours and who must therefore tailor their views to the demands of the social context' (Durrheim, 2012, p. 188). When one explores the variety and intensity of prejudices in society one cannot paper over the complex range of visible, accountable behaviours of social actors, and the role of institutional, legal, economic frameworks. It would be a mistake to relegate prejudice solely to the realm of implicit attitudes, to the unconscious (and automatic) workings of the individual mind. When one is interested in prejudice as a social problem, one cannot ignore social actions and social interactions, as well as social and symbolic frameworks of meaning-making.

One step in the right direction is made by studies that are trying to extend the notion of implicit prejudice to social interaction. Durrheim writes about socio-communicative situations where prejudiced attitudes and stereotypes are expressed in very subtle, implicit ways; what he calls 'stereotyping by implication'. These are situations in which stereotypical representations serve interpersonal as well as ideological functions (Durrheim, 2014). By stereotyping in non-categorical form or by using a vague reference or indirect association between people and social traits, offensive stereotyping can remain implicit. In their work on 'collaborative prejudice', Condor *et al.* (2006) and Condor and Figgou (2012) show how, in multi-party discussions, stereotypes or supposedly negative evaluations are 'socially occasioned', and how the expression of prejudice in interaction is carefully 'policed' by other members.

For both Durrheim and Condor and colleagues, a precise social and rhetorical context matters. As I will be showing in the next three chapters, this also matters for discursive psychologists. Prejudice is not lodged in the unconscious recesses of the minds of participants to interaction but in the immediate and broader conversational context elicited by the use of open-ended research methods (e.g. open-ended or semi-structured interviews). Speakers and hearers, co-participants, regulate the expression of prejudiced beliefs by facilitating or resisting, transforming, the open expression of (offensive) prejudices.

The prejudiced subject is a social being actively using cultural resources for justification and criticism (Billig, 1996). If, as Myrdal argues, 'stereotypes are ideological fragments which have been coined and sanctioned' (1996 [1944], p. 42) by the societies in which they find expression, then prejudices need to be studied as social and cultural creations. The intensity or subtlety, and direction, of prejudices may be affected by the level of social support/facilitation or resistance in social interactional contexts, as well as by the 'level of abstractness at which ... issues are talked about' (Figgou and Condor, 2006, p. 239). I will return to prejudice in interaction in the next chapters.

Social categorization and contexts of social identity

Implicit measures emphasize automatic and unconscious aspects and describe prejudice as an outcome of *natural* psychological processes, and not as a symbolic and contextual phenomenon. Yet, social experiences and the history of social relations between people show that the prejudiced subject is a social being that actively places their evaluations in a social context. A focus on implicit prejudiced attitudes only partly explains what Memmi called the tragic dilemma of racism in social life. What is the nature of the context in which people make their beliefs, feelings, attitudes (prejudiced or otherwise) accountable to others? If we consider people as participants in social relations that are not only physical but also symbolic, then it is not enough to describe what is going on in terms of implicit processing/evaluations of individuals and intergroup relations.

Implicit measures attest to the influence of what has been called 'methodological individualism', with 'theory and research focusing on isolated individuals' (Zerubavel and Smith, 2010, p. 324). We need to be able to place both implicit and explicit attitudes in collective contexts of symbolism and identity. When considering the predicament of Romani people in Europe this task becomes an urgent task.

Processes of categorization and stereotyping were taken a step further with social identity theory (Brown, 1995; Tajfel, 1981a; Tajfel and Turner, 1986) and self-categorization theory (Turner, 1999b; Turner *et al.*, 1987). It was a step forward from the individualistic limitations of cognition research to greater emphasis on the social context (Tajfel, 1981a) of group interaction and correlate issues of power, status, differentiation between social groups

(Billig, 1976; Tajfel, 1978). Although minimal group studies (Billig and Tajfel, 1973; Tajfel *et al.*, 1971) have shown how social categorization can inevitably produce discrimination, modern social psychology qualifies this emphasis by saying that discrimination is not an inevitable outcome of categorization, and that although categorization is necessary, it is not sufficient for discrimination (Tajfel and Turner, 1986).

Social identity theory (SIT) and self-categorization theory (SCT) have developed on two interrelated fronts. First, a cognitive front that kept intact all the assumptions regarding the basic processes of classification and categorization. Second, a motivational front, which started as a motivational theory of self-esteem, mainly from the idea that one's own self-worth is defined in the arena of intergroup comparisons. According to this, group members will be motivated to maximize the differences between groups by favouring the in-group, and emphasize the positive distinctiveness of their own group on any valued dimension.

The theoretical perspectives of SIT and SCT are structured and shaped by the encounter between the 'individual' and the 'social' (Reicher, 2004). For example, it was experimentally demonstrated that threats to people's social identities are responded to with attempts to differentiate the in-group positively from out-groups (e.g. Bourhis and Giles, 1977; Breakwell, 1978). It may happen nevertheless that similarity (whether of status or attitudes) may promote attraction between groups (Brewer and Campbell, 1976; Brown and Abrams, 1986). Issues related to the dynamics of the social identity of inferior groups, groups of subordinate status, were also approached experimentally. For example, Tajfel and Turner (1986) suggest that a possible response in cases of low self-esteem of subordinate group belonging is to abandon the current social identity or to find and promote different dimensions of comparison.

Developments in SCT have put forward new ways of thinking about intergroup phenomena. For example, Reynolds and Turner (2001) state that the 'progress in understanding "prejudice" requires recognition that it is a group process that originates in the psychology of the group, intergroup relations, and the reality of human social conflict' (p. 178). For the two authors, prejudice is not 'an outcome of irrationality, deficiency, and pathology, *it can be understood as a psychological rational and valid product of the way members of certain groups perceive the social structure of intergroup relations*' (ibid., emphasis in original). According to this, prejudices are the outcome of the 'rational selectivity of perception' (Turner, 1999b, p. 26). Thus, stereotyping does not 'impoverish, but enriches social perception' (ibid., p. 27). For Reynolds and Turner (2001), social antagonism, as a psychologically rational and valid[3] product of the way members of certain groups perceive the social structure of intergroup relations, '*arises from and reflects their subjectively-apprehended understanding of the relationships between groups in society*' (p. 160, emphasis in original).

Reynolds and Turner (2001) propose an alternative analysis of prejudice. The contention is that both prejudiced and unprejudiced groups are engaged 'in the *same psychology*' (p. 173, emphasis in original). Their perspective stems 'from the *same* categorization process in interaction with intergroup relations and social structural factors' (ibid., emphasis in original; see also Oakes and Haslam, 2001). But if both the oppressor and the oppressed are engaged in the same psychology, how can we distinguish between the various intensities and ideological importance of prejudices? How can we distinguish between subtle and blatant prejudices? How can we get out of the dilemma of the inevitability of prejudice?

Early versions of social identity and self-categorization theory constituted themselves as a theory of prejudice, keeping intact a 'tendency to universalise the conditions for racism and a lingering perceptualism' (Wetherell and Potter, 1992, p. 47; see also Billig, 2002a). According to this view, prejudices are either a matter of differentiation between groups, a problem of ethnocentrism that favours in-groups and denigrates out-groups, or an issue of a psychologically rational and valid product of the way members of certain groups perceive the social structure of intergroup relations. As theories of prejudice, social identity and self-categorization theory can only partly explain the cultural, historical and ideological specificities of prejudice, and fail to satisfactorily distinguish between prejudice and bigotry and elaborate on the possible continuum between depersonalization and dehumanization (Billig, 2002a, 2002b). As Billig argues, in order 'to understand the nature of bigotry, one needs to pay close attention to what bigots say and, in particular, to the ideology of bigotry' (Billig, 2002b, p. 202).[4]

Modern SIT has shifted from a theory of prejudice to a theory of group freedom, emancipation and mobilization (Reicher, 2012). As Billig argues,

> social identity theory is not a theory of prejudice ... It is, at root, a theory of group freedom. It tells of the way that oppressed groups can find ways to challenge groups that have the power to ascribe identities and stereotypes.
>
> (2002a, p. 179)

Reicher (2011, p. 391) captures very convincingly this new impetus:

> the social world comes to structure human actors through the dynamics of selfhood. This insight derives from re-thinking and problematizing the nature of the self and, hence, the nature of all self-related terms. Thus, we can no longer simply claim that people respond to events that are self-relevant, that their actions are moderated and motivated by matters of self-esteem, or (perhaps most profoundly) that they act in terms of self-interest.

Modern social identity theory extends and clarifies the core assumption of classic social identity theory that says that society is constructed and structured along the lines of discrete social categories in relations of power, status and prestige with one another (cf. Hogg and Abrams, 1988). Haslam and Reynolds (2012) labour this point when they argue that the potency of prejudice in society comes from three factors. First, prejudice is underpinned by shared social identity – 'socially potent forms of prejudice reflect *collective* understandings that are grounded in a particular model of social identity … group members come to *share* particular beliefs about both in-group and out-group that gives those beliefs their force' (p. 435, emphasis in original). What counts is the 'socially structured nature of prejudice' with practices of identity formation and resistance and 'identity' entrepreneurship as core dimensions. Second, prejudice is promoted through power and perceived vested interests that are the result of identity-based leadership and mobilization. Leaders, as entrepreneurs of identity, 'play a key role in actively crafting the meanings of social identity and the interpretations of intergroup relations that give rise to various forms of prejudice' (ibid.). Third, prejudice needs to be seen as political, not only as a purely psychological phenomenon. The political aspects of prejudice concern as much the collective views of the in-group as they do the out-group (Drury, 2012). Collective definitions, images, of oppressed groups can serve various identity-based functions, as well as ideological and system-justifying functions (see Dixon *et al.*, 2012).

These three aspects identified by Haslam and Reynolds do not operate in a social vacuum. They operate in specific argumentative contexts where social identities are mobilized, transformed or resisted. These social identities 'are implicated in processes that are critical in shaping and changing people's minds, motivations and behaviours' (Reynolds *et al.*, 2012, p. 55). These argumentative contexts of identity are public contexts (organizational, political, legal, etc.) where identity projects can take a variety of trajectories, and have anticipated as well as unanticipated consequences. In these argumentative contexts of identity categorization and identity construction takes the form of discursive and symbolic action.

Argumentative contexts of identity: categorization as discursive and symbolic action

The kinds of social categories people use to communicate about the social world reflect underlying ideological assumptions. Categories are important because they communicate something of the taken-for-granted, shared meanings that people have of the world. Categories define and control conceptions of reality. These conceptions can have both essentializing and de-essentializing effects (see Verkuyten, 2003), oppressive as well as progressive outcomes. These effects or outcomes cannot be determined in advance.

Some of the categories we use to describe individuals and groups have, sometimes, clear political and evaluative connotations (Augoustinos and Walker, 1998). Others are more ambiguous, and leave room for interpretation. Categories or identities are also a matter of debate depending on who is using them, and for what purpose. As Wetherell and Potter (1992) suggested, categorization works to 'catch' reality in discourse: 'the discursive act creates groups, interests, emotions, similarities and differences, a social landscape, an anthropology, a psychology of identity and even a geography' (p. 146). As a discursive act, categorization creates symbolic worlds and meanings where identities can latch on. As I argued earlier, if we fail to place implicit (as well as explicit) attitudes in collective contexts of symbolism and identity, then we will fail to understand the societal complexity of prejudices.

I consider descriptions of Romani identity in contemporary Europe to show how self- and other-categorizations and social identities are intimately linked and shaped in the context of social, and structural, relations between people (Okely, 2010).

Matras (2004) writes about and identifies a tension (and competition) between two opposing paradigms of Roma identity in the works of Barany (2002) and Hancock (2002). Both paradigms of Roma identity perpetuate *collective* understandings of social identity projects that are grounded in a particular model of identity entrepreneurship. In the first paradigm, that of Barany, the 'expert' uses an evidence-based framework to draw up a set of guidelines that would ultimately define how the Roma are to be described and treated. Symbolic aspects of what it means to be Roma/Gypsy are secondary. In the second paradigm, that of Hancock, the Roma themselves are ethnographic authorities on their own culture. Symbolic aspects of what it means to be Roma/Gypsy are primordial.

In the remainder of the chapter I show how, in the context of national Roma policy and/or cross-national issues of migration, lay and elite constructions of the Roma lead to quandaries or dilemmas of definition/categorization. In the context of an enlarged Europe, social identities can cause a great deal of anxiety by what they seem to conceal rather than by what they reveal (cf. Memmi, 2000). I also show how definitions/categorizations are intertwined with the ethnicization and de-ethnicization of Roma, and the symbolic aspects associated with these moves that lead to their exclusion and misrepresentation.

In a study of perceptions of Roma migrants in Austria, Benedik (2010) documents the shift from the general identity category 'Roma beggars' to more specific (gender and ethnic) descriptions of migrant Roma. Benedik identifies the conditions under which categorization changes over time, leading to the creation of new categories. He shows how the recategorization of Roma serves very specific social functions linked to perceptions and elite management of social cohesion and solidarity. As Benedik argues, between 1989 and 1996, it was unclear to residents what category of people were doing the begging. Although 'beggars' originated from Slovakia, ex-Yugoslavia and other places, the category 'Roma' was used as a general label. The term 'beggar' (and by implication, Roma) was associated with 'vagrancy' or 'troublemaking'. However, once more public information became available the category 'beggars' was differentiated from other categories linked to public order and control. Once more information about the 'background' of 'beggars' became shared knowledge and started to circulate actively in private and public spheres, descriptions became more specific: 'beggars from abroad' (that is, 'poor' countries from the European 'East') (cf. Benedik, 2010).[5] A more concrete picture of the 'beggars' made reference to their 'gender'. As Benedik notes, this apparent move of de-ethnicization allowed for a more flexible definition of begging as a practice: a distinction was introduced between 'acceptable' (young men from Slovakia) and 'unacceptable' (women and their children from ex-Yugoslavia) ways of begging. Women (and their children) were portrayed as engaged in 'aggressive' begging, whereas begging by a (young) man was considered acceptable. Gendered begging not only had implications for understanding the practice of begging but also had consequences for understanding the *kind* of people that were doing the begging (and their values). One of the negative consequences of gendering begging was the proliferation of private and public perceptions of (dysfunctional family) Roma culture.

Ethnographic studies, such as Benedik's, can reveal the social complexity, and transformative nature, of social categorizations and descriptions of people, and the contextual-relational nature of identity categories (see also Okely, 1983). The contextual-relational nature of identity categories cannot be simply inferred from the social context in which they operate, or are created. The contextual-relational nature of identity categories is more an upshot of the flexible, and continuous, interaction between a specific social context, public flows of information, and social and political priorities.

For instance, in the context of managing intra-European migration, European countries have to justify the treatment they reserve for 'newcomers' in terms of either ethnicization or de-ethnicization of ethnic categories to which these newcomers are seen to belong. For example, France failed to uphold its state policy against ethnicization by referring explicitly to the Roma as an ethnic group. As Nacu (2012) argues, 'among the things which shocked observers was the explicit way in which the Roma were referred to as an ethnic group, which, until recently, was unusual in public debate for those sharing the general democratic consensus' (p. 1326). Its policies were directed at the Roma *because* they were identified, in the first place, as Roma. Although French legislation prohibits explicit use of ethnic identification and upholds the values of equal treatment and freedom of movement and settlement, this did not stop the French police from issuing a memo calling for the 'systematic' eviction of Roma from temporary, and supposedly illegal, camps, on the basis of their ethnicity.[6] Interestingly, in Italy, a different move, of de-ethnicization, was used to justify the harassment of European citizens of Roma origin. The Italian Minister of the Interior, Roberto Maroni (cited by Stewart, 2012b), claimed in 2010 that the collection of personal data (fingerprinting) of young people living in 'nomad camps' was not about the Roma, but 'only about nomad camps'. As such, it could not be construed as an 'ethnicity-based measure' but a response to a 'de facto situation', the presence of the 'unauthorized nomad camps'. By avoiding the label 'Roma' or 'Gypsy' the Italian authorities inoculated themselves against charges of discrimination based on ethnic origin. Okely (1983) has documented similar de-ethnicization practices in 1960s Britain that helped with the introduction of harsher legislation and were used to avoid or manage accusations of racism and discrimination. As Okely argues, non-ethnic 'definitions' of Gypsies (as a person 'leading a nomadic life ... with no fixed abode') were used to rewrite some legislation to make it difficult to challenge pieces of legislation such as the Highways Act or Caravan Sites Act.

Both ethnicized and de-ethnicized categories such as 'nomads' permit the creation of a order of worth, and dignity, in society. The 'settled', the 'civilized', have the right, and power, to alter, to transform the dignity and social form of life of others who are considered unworthy. The use of ethnicized and de-ethnicized categories makes one forget that 'Gypsy culture inhabits and constructs its internal coherence alongside or in opposition to other dominating cultures; in the same geographical and political space' (Okely, 2010, p. 40).

Of course, there may be occasions where the ethnicization of the Roma may have positive consequences (such as protecting them, as Roma, from discriminatory state measures by making them more visible). Or cases where de-ethnicization moves lead to an extension of identity categories that might include a wider platform of definition – not only in terms of ethnicity, but also gender, occupation, personal history, etc. What both ethnicization and de-ethnicization practices show is that there is a considerable dimension of mobilization in prejudice. As Reicher argues, 'wherever we find prejudice, it has been mobilized, it has been mobilized deliberately and it has been mobilized for gain' (2012, p. 30). Prejudice is mobilized by elites, through legal systems, the media, etc. When one considers examples of ethnicization and de-ethnicization, one comes to appreciate perhaps more clearly the limitations of a perspective on prejudice that considers prejudice as a feature of implicit, unconscious or automatic individual cognition. These examples show that the classic prejudiced mind is a social mind; it is not just the mind of ordinary members of society 'perceiving' negative qualities in others, but also the mind of an elite that mobilizes prejudice for strategic social and political gains.[7]

Mobilizing prejudice for strategic social and political gain carries symbolic weight. For instance, as Fraser argues, 'the meanings attached to the term "Gypsy" ... a semantic problem not of the Gypsies' making' (1992, p. 1). The Roma/Gypsies are usually talked about in terms of their social identity as 'Roma' or 'Gypsies', and not in terms of personal identity. They are talked about by virtue of membership to a specific social category. The categories used by others to talk about the Roma do not have anything corresponding in the Romani language (the Roma's own frame of reference). The French word 'tsigane' is not a word in Romani and is not associated with anything precise in Roma's frame of reference; instead it corresponds to a symbolic representation replete with positive and negative connotations. Social identities do not solely reflect the cognitive and emotional significance of belonging to groups, but also reflect symbolic aspects. If social identities only 'represent the group-based aspect of the self' (Reynolds *et al.*, 2012, p. 56), how can we account for how people respond to symbolism embedded in identities, as the case of Roma in Europe shows?

The history of expressions of hostility makes reference to the symbolism of social and identity categories. In *Portrait of a Jew*, Memmi (1963) paints the portrait of the imaginary (mythical) Jew, which includes (but is not limited to) what he calls the 'misfortune of being a Jew'. 'Being a Jew' presupposes biological/perceptual frames as well as symbolic and mythical aspects. In the same way, one can talk of the misfortune of being Roma/Gypsy. Media reports perpetuate, recycle, ancient myths of child kidnapping/stealing (see the recent high-profile case of Maria, the 'blond angel' supposedly 'abducted' by a family of Gypsies), sexual promiscuity, lying, thieving, wild passion, etc. Romani social identity symbolism is a very complex phenomenon.

As Kligman argues, 'Gypsies or Roma … are simultaneously among history's most romanticized and reviled of peoples' (2001, p. 62). They are 'both seductive and feared' (ibid.). For example, a recent investigation into the portrayal of 'the Gypsy woman' at the Museum of the Romanian Peasant in Bucharest (Hasdeu, 2008, p. 350) has revealed how the Museum

> uncritically reproduces extremely entrenched and widespread pan-European representations which place peasants and Gypsies in opposition. On the whole, the representation of Gypsies constructed by the Museum reinforces the stereotypical idea that Gypsies belong to an orgiastic space–time out of line with normality.

As Hasdeu argues, the museum makes the most of symbolic Gypsy stereotypes to 'project an image that is oneiric, absurd and carnivalesque, and it does so at least in part through the utilisation of women and images of femininity' (ibid., p. 356).

The cultural image of the Gypsy points to an inadaptable essence of foreign and exotic origin and culture. As Okely argues, 'the threat which the Gypsies, as a minority, appear to represent to the larger society is largely ideological' (1983, p. 213). They defy the dominant societal systems of education, labour and employment. This leads nation-states to attempt to manage them through policies that embed, to various degrees, 'condescension and impatience, ... paternalism and despotism, ... benevolent inactivity and strenuous attempts at radical solutions' (Fraser, 1992, p. 277).

> The Roms are often depicted as a group that likes to isolate itself from the mainstream. While it is of course true that many Romani people are protective of their culture and values, they are also a model of cultural tolerance and flexibility. They are traditionalists who maintain ancient customs. Yet at the same time they are reformers who do not resist ideas and practices simply because they were introduced by others, but embrace them and integrate them into their lives.
>
> (Matras, 2014, p. 227)

Regardless of the complexity of Romani identity, Romani people are portrayed as carriers of immutable cultural essences, especially when they are romanticized. For instance, what Okely (1983) calls the romance of 'foreign origin' and 'exotic culture' undermines Romani people's right to self-determination. Romanticized images call Romani people to account for their existence in terms other than their own.

Romani 'nomadism' is another symbolic aspect at the heart of the social representation of the group (Moscovici, 2011). The multiplicity of Roma identities and alternative ways of life are downplayed because of the influence, and social and political perpetuation, of the nomadism myth (Asséo, 1994). Nomadism (as well as sedentarism) carries symbolic import. For instance, descriptions of Roma/Gypsies as indigenous groups – in Transylvania (Olivera, 2012) or Greece (Zachos, 2011) – are very different (at a symbolic level) from descriptions of the new European nomadism (see also Stewart, 2012b on various other descriptions of nomadism and sedentarism across the world). Symbolism is revealed in practices of labelling and conflicting labels being applied to people. The example of Kosovar Roma in Italy is a cogent one as it shows how different types of labelling/categorization ('nomads' or 'refugees') have different social consequences for the Roma so labelled (Sigona, 2003). When one is classed as a 'nomad' one is presented as a certain type of person, with less entitlement to social services and protection under the law than when one is classed as a 'refugee'. However, regardless of whether they are categorized as 'nomads' or 'refugees', the Roma 'do not exist as individuals for the Italian public but only as stereotypes ... many Roma have effectively been forced to live out the romantic, but repressive, projections of Italians' (ibid., p. 76).

Intracommunity categorization, self-definition and affirmation

Throughout their history, Roma have been forced to shape their subjectivity out of images, symbols and metaphors provided and used by more powerful others. This is a state of affairs deplored by some Roma activists. Roma activists talk of being a 'gypsy' as the worst stigma (Valeriu Nicolae on Romania), and deplore the ambiguity of the identity projects of the European Union that do not recognize the diversity of the Roma.

> Discussions on the Roma at the European level are plagued by ambiguities, as is the very question of Roma identity itself. Roma are lumped together by national governments, intergovernmental institutions and civil society in a comfortable paradigm that blatantly contradicts the well-acknowledged fact that there are numerous groups of Roma that have very little in common with each other. A large number of Roma groups have very different traditions, languages, religions and lifestyles.
>
> (Nicolae, 2012)

Roma's own images of themselves shape a different kind of subjectivity. Identity categories are not only *negatively* defined by the prejudiced gaze of the majority, but are also *positively* defined by the tensions of self-definition. The symbolic image capital of the Roma is the result of these two processes, with different effects depending on the social context.

The categories used by Roma/Gypsies to define themselves testify to the variety of experiences of 'being Roma/Gypsy', of 'realising Gypsyness' (Horvath, 2012, p. 127). Ethnographic research has pointed out the variety of intracommunity categorizations and descriptions that set Roma/Gypsies apart from one another. Horvath (2012) shows a very detailed system of in-group differentiation amongst Roma in Hungary. Those who resided in cave-dwellings were seen as 'dirty' and showing 'exaggerated Gypsiness' ('showing off'). Those living in houses were considered 'fussy', and seen as 'pretending to be Hungarians'. In contrast to the Hungarian 'other', 'the Hungarian environment was a condition perceived as constant, it was the frame into which the Gypsy had to fit, or towards which one had to adapt in order to get by' (ibid., p. 131). As Csepeli and Simon (2004) also argue, 'the Gypsy-image of the majority is more or less homogenous, stereotypical and fraught with negative bias, while the self-image of the Roma is heterogeneous' (p. 129).

Other studies (cf. Durst, 2010) document the heterogeneous Roma self-image, and the range of identity categories used by Gypsies themselves for intragroup differentiation – 'mobile' Gypsies, assimilated Gypsies ('white' Gypsies), 'slum-dweller' Gypsies. As Durst argues, the social meaning of 'being a Gypsy' differs according to locality and human condition: 'being a Gypsy is something totally different for the assimilated stratum from Lapos, for the "slum-dwellers" of the same village or for the Roma inhabitants of Paloca' (ibid., p. 27). Ethnographic research has also shown how various Roma groups can choose different dimensions of social comparison in order to operate intragroup distinctions. For instance, the Transylvanian Gabori distinguish themselves from other Roms, and present themselves as 'hard-working' and 'civilized', and as having an occupation (e.g. coppersmiths) transmitted through generations of Roma.

Such a varied basis for definition can create problems for researchers that rely on Roma/Gypsy social identification for research or census purposes. Who is Roma/Gypsy and who is not is a frequent quandary that survey researchers, for instance, have to face. As some researchers argue (Csepeli and Simon, 2004; Rughiniş, 2012), different methods of classification can elicit different results in studies of the Roma. What researchers find is that, although 'the experience of being Roma is determined by the convergence of factors such as ancestry, mother tongue, neighbourhood, and social bonds', even 'in the absence of the entirety of these factors, it still is possible to be categorised, by the outgroup, as Roma' (Csepeli and Simon, 2004, p. 138). Perceptual frames such as skin colour or social aspects such as family name or speech can be used to draw a type-portrait of Roma, but actual identity categorization can vary quite starkly, depending on local or national context and the nature of identity elicitation techniques (interviews, surveys, etc.). Moreover, as Csepeli and Simon (2004) note, 'the tendency to self-identify with the Roma community is also far from universal' (p. 148) across a variety of contexts. It is not only researchers but also European institutions that are having difficulties in 'defining' Romani identity. According to Matras, 'we find an array of contradictory labels and definitions employed in the media and popular speech, as well as in legal documents and political resolutions' (2014, p. 20). Matras emphasizes the difficulty that official documents have in defining the Roma, alluding ambiguously to groups with different appellations sharing 'more or less similar cultural characteristics' (Open Society Institute, 2011).

Ethnographic studies of Romani identity support some of the findings of social psychological research on the flexibility and context-dependent constructions of identity (cf., for example, Merino and Tileagă, 2011; Verkuyten and deWolf, 2002). But they also add a very important anthropological (and symbolic) dimension to understanding self-definition. They highlight the anthropological and symbolic significance of self-definition for identity construction (Okely, 1983), and the strategic nature of self-ascriptions.

Romani people are strategic entrepreneurs of identity, adapting continuously to the ideology of the dominant society, 'picking up some things, rejecting others' (Okely, 1983, p. 77). Strategic differentiation lies at the core of Romani identity. Individual and group identity is defined in relation to a shifting social context. Romani historian Sarah Carmona, cited by *The New Yorker*, captures the strategic nature of Romani identity and some of its consequences for dominant groups:

> We can be Roma in the political sphere, be considered Sinti in another, family sphere. We can even become Gypsies, tsiganes, in order to deal

> with non-Roma people. This is a traumatic topic for official thought. Imagine: a people multiple in themselves, not in solidarity with us.
>
> (Gopnik, 2014)

There is much about Roma/Gypsy culture and way of being in the world that is concealed from non-Gypsies, aspects that reinforce ethnic boundaries: for example, 'pollution beliefs' – eating, washing, the use of space and the use/placing of objects in space (Okely, 1983), assumptions about the body, food and health, spatial organization, animal symbolism, etc. (see Okely, 1983 and Matras, 2014 for brilliant accounts of the link between everyday practices and complex identity symbolism).[8]

In their exploration of natural categorizations of Romanies in Czech television debates, Leudar and Nekvapil (2000) reveal how 'facts' about Roma as a culturally unique form of life were only known, and used, by Roma themselves, to justify and counter negative stereotyping. Ethnographies show that performances of social identity can be limited by 'strong and rigid' boundaries between groups (Horvath, 2012). In the context of Gypsy life in an Hungarian village, Horvath shows how Gypsy identity is more likely to be performed in private but not in public. In the public sphere, the label 'Gypsy' (and people labelled as 'Gypsies') had a clearly inferior and subordinate 'place' in the school, workplaces, public places, in the village. However, the meaning of 'Gypsy' in the village was nonetheless subject to transformation. For instance, the 'Gypsyness' of Gypsy children became more relevant when attempts were made to integrate them into the local school. Hungarian children gradually left as their parents moved them to a different school. A 'Gypsy' NGO-led programme of transforming the Gypsy settlements made the 'Gypsy' voice more relevant, yet the local Hungarians perceived this as a 'brutal breach of the old order, as a kind of loss of territory' (ibid., p. 120). Interestingly, even after attempts to make it more visible, more 'respectable', Gypsy identity was only reluctantly used in public 'as an openly assumed collective experience or as a collective resource' (ibid., p. 124).

The failure to recognize Romani people as embodying 'respectable' identities modifies their perceived worth. An identity category (such as 'Gypsy', 'Roma') that, in private, is a resource for self-affirmation and self-definition is, in public, a resource for self-degradation, that justifies social and moral exclusion.

Romani people are more likely to be described as living on the edge of poverty or using romanticized images than in terms of 'respectable' (professional or community-related) identities: 'community leader', 'businessperson', 'politician', 'law-abiding citizen'. As Blackwood *et al.* argue,

> identity is not simply important as a way of looking at oneself and looking at the world. It also has real consequences for what we can do. To

> be denied an identity is to be denied a position from which one can act upon the world.
>
> (2013, p. 1101)

Failure to be recognized in terms that are consistent with how individual, groups or communities see (or would like to see) themselves can have pernicious consequences for securing a position from which to 'act upon the world'. One can be shifted, interrogated, evicted, etc., on the basis of ascribed identities. Where strong subjective meanings of identity, such as those of the Roma, are not taken into account, one relegates people to a lesser degree of dignity.

The paradoxical promise that liberal, democratic societies make to the Roma is that they will be treated fairly but only on the condition that they slowly, but surely, abandon their separate identity and way of life (Matras, 2014). Romani activism, and affirmation of ethnic identity, is encouraged only to the extent that it supports the declared inclusionary goals of European societies that force Romani people to gradually abandon their diverse ways of self-definition and their idea of common belonging (what Romani people call *Romanipen*). Interestingly, Romani activism and/or political mobilization are not perceived as a threat. As Sigona and Trehan (2009, p. 8) argue,

> unsurprisingly, the neoliberal gaze on Roma privileges spaces and forms of political mobilization which are ultimately 'safe' because they do not pose a threat to the assumptions on which the neoliberal order rests, and hence do not confront nor address the structural causes of the socio-economic marginality that affects the vast majority of Romani communities.

The neoliberal gaze on Romani identity privileges forms of identity that influence, directly or indirectly, the dialogue about the moral status that should be assigned to the Roma in European societies. Discursive and symbolic categorizations and assumptions mobilized in a variety of argumentative contexts of identity define different degrees and intensities of worth, respect and dignity of people. The mobilization of discursive and symbolic categorizations and assumptions also shows that prejudice is not only a matter of psychological (automatic, implicit) appraisals or evaluations but also a matter of people's (discursive and symbolic) practices in specific social contexts. Other- and self-definitions, tolerant and intolerant worldviews, take their power and significance from the identity contexts in which they are mobilized. They also possess a highly visible social and rhetorical complexity steeped in *ways of talking* that combine, to different degrees, compassionate, paternalistic, conflictual, dehumanizing and eliminationist repertoires. I turn to the analysis of these ways of talking in the next three chapters.

Notes

1 Social cognition marks a shift from understanding prejudices in terms of personality structure to understanding prejudices based on misinformation, bias, cognitive distortion and the need to keep the cognitive load to a minimum. And yet, there are two presuppositions that are common to both personality and social cognition approaches: 'the belief in rationality as an ideal for democratic society and the emphasis on the individual as the site of the breakdown of this rationality and therefore as the object of research' (Henriques, 1984, p. 66).
2 According to Hewstone *et al.* (2002), the notion of 'bias' can 'encompass behavior (discrimination), attitude (prejudice) and cognition (stereotyping)' (p. 576). They argue that the use of the term 'bias' 'involves an interpretative judgment that the response is unfair, illegitimate, or unjustifiable, in the sense that it goes beyond the objective requirements or evidence of the situation' (ibid.).
3 As Billig (2002a) suggests, part of self-categorization research is devoted to exploring the extent to which stereotyping might be 'veridical'. It is worth noting that Billig places this kind of work as being antithetical to the work of Henri Tajfel (see Augoustinos and Walker, 1998 for a critique of research that attempts to conceptualize stereotypes as accurate or veridical).
4 I return to Billig's point in Chapter 7 when discussing extreme prejudice and dehumanization as discursive actions.
5 As Benedik shows, the ethnicization of Roma as beggars had mixed results. On the one hand, it raised public awareness regarding their fate (especially after a tragic event). On the other hand, it opened the way for the negative stereotyping of Roma as beggars, and the return of racist discourses in the press.
6 Following an outcry from Roma rights organizations and human rights watchdogs the memo was 'rectified', although evictions have continued (see Amnesty International, 2014).
7 Elites 'do not mobilize prejudice by accident or by chance' (Reicher, 2012, p. 38). Ensuring compliance with the rules and norms of the majority, instituting social order, requires the mobilization of identity categories that alter or transform people's worth.
8 In this symbolic world (sometimes known only to the Roma), authenticity plays an important part. In what Matras (2014) calls the 'mosaic' of Romani groups, 'each Gypsy grouping tends to look upon itself as being the authentic Gypsies' (Fraser, 1992, p. 8).

Chapter 5

The discourse of prejudice

Racism as discursive ideology

Discourse analysis and researching prejudice as social problem

As I argued in Chapter 1, European societies are engaged in a dialogue about the moral status that should be assigned to the Roma. This dialogue is conducted in the public and cultural spheres and media, but also in everyday conversations. This dialogue is driven by elite and lay ways of talking that allow members of European societies to define different degrees and intensities of worth, respect and dignity for Romani people. These ways of talking can combine tolerant, compassionate, paternalistic, conflictual, dehumanizing and eliminationist repertoires. They span the political spectrum. These ways of talking show that it is possible for common perceptions of Roma's subhumanity to coexist with benevolent attitudes. Understanding these ways of talking is essential to understanding the (societal) mechanism of assigning, transforming or altering Romani people's worth and dignity.

Although one can document expressions of direct hostility or attributions of extreme negative qualities to Roma in text and talk, a closer inspection shows that anti-Roma prejudice is much more complex. If, as I argued, we conceive of liberal democracies as an embodiment of modes of domination as well as empowerment/sympathy (Fassin, 2005), then we should be able to identify and analyse the nature of prejudices that emerge from this conception of society.

In this chapter I outline the contribution of discourse analysis in social psychology and linguistics to understanding racism as a discursive ideology. I contend that, when used appropriately, discourse analysis can make a valuable contribution to a deeper understanding of the collective social conditions that make both tolerance and intolerance possible (Tileagă, 2014).

Discourse analysis can help our understanding of how talk and text about social problems is suffused with rhetorical complexity. By proposing a methodological stance that respects the nature of the empirical world (Blumer, 1998 [1969]), the discourse analysis of contrived and naturally occurring data (semi-structured interviews, focus groups, media texts, public debates) sourced in the complex social imaginary of societies can be a potent way into understanding the various meaning-making practices through which both tolerance and intolerance are organized and operate in society.

Racism in general, and anti-Roma racism in particular, possesses a highly visible social and rhetorical complexity. However, social psychologists routinely portray it as an outcome of responsive or passive psychological modes. Whenever racism is measured through implicit or explicit measures, it is stripped of its rhetorical, ideological and societal intricacies. In this chapter I want to highlight how racism operates in argumentative spaces of ideology, and how (racist) attitudes, views, positions, etc., possess marked rhetorical complexity (Billig, 1996; Gamson, 1992; Lane, 1962). I also argue that, although discourse analysis offers a solid and promising epistemological and methodological apparatus that can contribute successfully to fulfilling the main goal of a critical analysis of racism, it can only partially engage with the different societal nuances of racism unless it is placed in a broader critical analytic framework. As argued in Chapter 1, the main goal of a critical analysis of racism is to understand the operative social practices and societal principles that regulate processes of inclusion and exclusion and the argumentative spaces, ways of talking, they generate and feed upon.

Discourse and prejudice

The crux and focus of discourse-analytic approaches to the language of prejudice is aptly described by Michael Billig:

> it would seem to be more profitable to relate prejudice to language, for the possession of linguistic skills is a necessary condition for the possession of prejudiced beliefs ... the expression of prejudiced attitudes is not some sort of epiphenomenon, but constitutes a central component of prejudice.
>
> (1985, p. 85)

One of the first systematic discourse-analytic attempts to 'map' prejudiced discourse was conducted by Uta Quasthoff (1978, 1989). Quasthoff distinguishes between 'attitudes', 'convictions' and 'prejudices' and sees 'stereotypes' as a typical element of verbally expressed common knowledge about group belonging. According to Quasthoff the outward expression of prejudices in the form of stereotypes functions socially as a means of phatic communion and also as a way of simplifying communication with the in-group and delineating the out-group (Quasthoff, 1989; see also Reisigl and Wodak, 2001). However, Quasthoff's explorations of the social function of prejudices and stereotypes do not transcend the sentence level. Other, earlier discourse-analytic studies – in the strand of research known as critical linguistics (Fowler *et al.*, 1979; Kress and Hodge, 1979) – emphasizes the role of grammatical, semantic and syntactic structures in the reproduction of dominance, power and control in discourse. For example, Fowler *et al.*'s (1979) seminal work on the role of power and control in language includes an analysis of a press coverage of an 'ethnic' event (the disturbances at the Notting Hill Carnival in London). Fowler *et al.* show how the syntactic structure of the sentences reflected the 'white' dominant perspective of the journalists, and how active and passive agency and responsibility for actions was managed through the use of passive forms and was emphasized syntactically. The study of Sykes (1985) about discrimination in discourse comes to similar conclusions involving the role of grammatical form in the textual presentation of 'us' and 'them'.

Teun van Dijk takes the importance of grammatical and syntactic features in the textual presentation of 'us' and 'them' to a different level, by embedding linguistic analysis in a socio-cognitive framework. In a series of innovative studies, van Dijk examined the ways in which majority group members in the Netherlands and the United States talk about minorities and ethnic relations in everyday conversations, the press and parliament and elite discourse (van Dijk, 1984, 1987, 1991, 1993). In van Dijk's work, the construction of 'difference' is accomplished through the combination of two key discursive strategies: 'positive self-presentation' and 'negative other-presentation'. These strategies operate alongside a range of more specific discursive resources used to rationalize prejudice against minority groups. As van Dijk *et al.* argue,

> at all levels of discourse, this overall principle will remain the same, namely a strategy that combines positive self-presentation with negative other-presentation. Obviously, it is this strategy that plays a primary role in the sociocognitive function of discourse about others, namely the formation of negative cognitions (specific mental models of concrete events, as well as more general group prejudices and ideologies) about outgroups.
>
> (1997, p. 166)

According to van Dijk, what we call 'discrimination' can be described by pointing to several discursive resources and strategies ('the 7 D's of discrimination'): dominance, differentiation, distance, diffusion, diversion, depersonalization and daily discrimination (cf. van Dijk, 1984). What psychologists would routinely describe in psychological terms – 'distance', 'differentiation' or 'depersonalization' – are analysed as linguistic expressions, discursive moves in social interaction. van Dijk has tried to link the expression of prejudice to the flexible and active use of discursive units larger than the sentence. He also explored 'preferred' types of issues involved in describing 'others' (such as deviance, difference and threat) in storytelling and narrative organization. For instance, the detailed discursive analysis of prejudiced stories reveals the role of rhetorical devices such as apparent denials, apparent admissions or apparent concessions (van Dijk, 1987, 1992). Although van Dijk shows the subtlety of verbal prejudice, where denials are only 'apparent', as prejudice continues to be upheld and reproduced discursively, he also writes about the role of semantic and episodic memory, as well as the role of schematic knowledge and group schemata in the explanation of the socio-cognitive dynamic of ethnic prejudice. According to van Dijk, discursive structures, underpinned by cognitive structures, ensure the perpetuation of racism in society.

For other researchers, racism is about the discursive enactment of power and domination in socio-historical context and perspective. As part of an extended and laborious programme of critical discourse studies, Ruth Wodak and her colleagues from the University of Vienna have explored the social, political and historical dimensions of anti-Semitic discourse in Austria (Wodak and Matouschek, 1993; see also Fairclough and Wodak, 1997). Wodak and colleagues are the proponents of a discourse-historical approach to the rhetoric of racism and anti-Semitism. As Wodak and Reisigl (1999) argue, the discourse-historical approach should be seen as an extension of van Dijk's socio-cognitive model (see also Mitten and Wodak, 1993). This discourse-analytical approach to the study of prejudice and racism is based on a more context-sensitive approach, including, amongst other dimensions of context, the broader socio-political and historical context, but also the history of the discursive practices that reproduce dominance. The discourse-historical analytic approach has been applied in a series of studies (de Cillia *et al.*, 1999; Wodak *et al.*, 1999) that have documented historical and contemporary content of discourses with racist, nationalist or anti-Semitic connotations. The discourse-historical approach has not only confirmed the complexity of prejudiced discursive patterns, but has also suggested that the prejudicial content that expressions of prejudice transmit is largely determined by the historical and linguistic contexts of their emergence (cf. Mitten and Wodak, 1993).

The work undertaken in social psychology in Britain by Michael Billig and colleagues (Billig, 1985; Billig *et al.*, 1988; Cochrane and Billig, 1984; Condor, 1988; Potter and Wetherell, 1987) was also a firm step to establish discourse analysis as a useful tool in the analysis of prejudice and racism. The work of Margaret Wetherell and Jonathan Potter on the language of racism in New Zealand (Wetherell and Potter, 1992) has also been of central importance in showing how discourse analysis can be used to question unequal relations of power and document the reproduction of dominance through talk. What is now known as 'discursive psychology' (see, for general outlines, Augoustinos and Tileagă, 2012; Edwards and Potter, 1992; Hepburn and Wiggins, 2007; Tileagă and Stokoe, in press) established an analytic trend that attempted to go beyond the semantic, pragmatic, grammatical and propositional levels of analysis advocated by socio-cognitive linguistic approaches.

For example, as van Dijk (1987) put it, 'talk about ethnic groups involves complex strategies and moves aiming at positive self-presentation within the overall of negative other-description' (p. 22). When delicate topics are under discussion, and when social norms are rather strict, he contended, face saving is essential. As he goes on to argue, 'the expression of even the most racist opinions tends to be embedded in moves that are intended to prevent the inference that the speaker is a racist' (ibid.). In discussing van Dijk, Billig (1988) claims that the assumption of a contradiction between racist attitudes and interactional strategies should be seen as a contradiction within the different ideological themes people draw upon. Billig *et al.* (1988) suggests that common sense is dilemmatic and people possess contrary themes as part of their commonsensical stock of knowledge. The argumentative nature of attitudes is also stressed, as attitudes are not merely linguistic moves, but represent stances in a matter of controversy (Billig, 1996). People are not solely concerned with positive self-presentation. The rhetorical context of attitudes implies that people will justify their stance and criticize competing views. As Billig *et al.* put it, 'beyond the issue of self-presentation there is an argumentative or rhetorical dimension. If views are to be presented as being rational and unprejudiced, then they must be seen to be justified, or at least to be justifiable' (1988, p. 113). Although discourse-analytic approaches in linguistics and social psychology may not share all fundamental presuppositions, they do nonetheless agree on a central point: that discourse is the 'prominent way in which ethnic prejudices and racism are reproduced in society' (van Dijk *et al.*, 1997, p. 144). Racist attitudes are seen as interpretative effects of descriptions and explanations (Potter and Wetherell, 1988; van Dijk, 1984, 1987; Wetherell and Potter, 1992). People use language to do things with words, to construct versions of the world (Potter and Wetherell, 1987) depending upon the function and orientation of their talk. Talk or text becomes a topic in its own right. As many other, more recent investigations have shown, constructions of tolerance and denials of feelings of prejudice are part of the common identity work of contemporary racist discourse (LeCouteur and Augoustinos, 2001; Tileagă, 2005).

Discourse (analysis) and ideology

Linguistic and social psychological discourse-analytic studies of racism have not only been concerned with the identification of discursive strategies or resources people use to express or discount prejudice. They have also offered a reinterpretation of the notion of 'ideology'. In this section I will briefly consider the different conceptualizations of ideology in discourse-analytic studies belonging to different disciplines and schools of thought. The turn to discourse in the social sciences has marked (and facilitated) a more general shift from a theory of ideology traditionally concerned with consciousness ('false consciousness') and processes of mystification of reality to a theory of ideology in terms of discursive performance. This came to the forefront with an awareness of the idea that 'ideology … concerns the actual uses of language between particular human subjects for the production of specific effects' (Eagleton, 1991, p. 9). Ideology is a discursive or semiotic phenomenon, is '"performative" rather than "constative" language: it belongs to the class of speech acts which get something done' (ibid., p. 19). Discourse is the site where (social) representations, interpretative repertoires and discursive resources are brought together in order to build a 'worldview' of social antagonism and unequal distribution of power. In other words, discourse is the site for the enactment of power, for reproducing dominance and inequality. As Paul Ricoeur argues,

> ideology is not the distortion of communication, but the rhetoric of basic communication. There is a rhetoric of human communication because we cannot exclude rhetorical devices from language; they are an intrinsic part of ordinary language. In its function as integration, ideology is similarly basic and ineluctable.
>
> (1986, p. 259)

As a consequence, it was considered more helpful to view ideology 'less as a particular *set* of discourses, than as a particular set of effects *within* discourses' (Eagleton, 1991, p. 194, italics in original). Ideological power, as John B. Thompson suggests, is not just a matter of meaning, but 'to make meaning stick' (1984, p. 132). Discourse-analytic approaches propose that racism be analysed not simply as a matter of linguistic or semantic practice, but also as a matter of discursive ideologies embedded in social and institutional practices, discriminatory actions and presuppositions about society (Wetherell and Potter, 1992).

Van Dijk (1998) proposes a theoretical framework for the study of ideology and discourse that critically relates discourse, cognition and society. In a nutshell, van Dijk sees ideologies as mental systems that organize socially shared attitudes. If emancipatory, liberal, arguments can be used in a discriminatory way, then it is the discriminatory effect of discourse that must be regarded as the main criterion for making discourses discernible as prejudiced or racist (Reisigl and Wodak, 2001; Wetherell and Potter, 1992). According van Dijk, the importance of studying ideology (or ideologies) arises from the belief that ideologies constitute the basis of social (cultural) representations shared by members of a group. As part of a socially shared belief system ideologies are both cognitive and social and they fulfil social and cognitive functions.

Other linguistically inspired approaches to issues of ideology centre on notions such as language and power (e.g. Fairclough, 1989) or the Gramscian notion of 'hegemony' (Chouliaraki and Fairclough, 1999). For Fairclough, ideologies are 'tied to action' and therefore need to be 'judged in terms of their social effects rather than their truth values' (1995, p. 76). Discursive practices are not ideological in themselves, but they are 'ideologically invested in so far as they incorporate significations which contribute to sustaining or restructuring power relations' (1992, p. 91). Fairclough's position is similar to that of Thompson (1984, 1990), that certain uses of language and other 'symbolic forms' are ideological, namely those which serve to establish or sustain relations of dominance. As Thompson emphasizes, '*to study ideology is to study the ways in which meaning serves to sustain relations of domination*' (1987, p. 519, italics in original). Ideologies embedded in discursive practices are most effective when they become naturalized, and achieve the status of 'common sense' (Fairclough, 1992).

Ruth Wodak and colleagues favour a context-sensitive approach to ideology. Amongst other dimensions of context, the context that Wodak and colleagues refer to is the

> broader sociopolitical and historical context which the discursive practices are embedded in and related to; that is to say, the fields of action and the history of the discursive event as well as the history to which the discourse topics are related.
>
> (Reisigl and Wodak, 2001, p. 41)

According to this view, the use of language presupposes the enactment of power, control and domination in a historical perspective. The articulation of ideologies in discourse is done through the enactment of different discursive practices with different ideological effects. Racist or anti-Semitic beliefs and ideologies are expressed and used for different aims. These have historical traditions and multiple roots. It is believed that through discourse analysis one is able 'to make explicit the whole range of linguistic devices used to code such beliefs and ideologies as well as the related practices' (Reisigl and Wodak, 2001, p. 266).

Social psychologists take a different approach to the analysis of ideology in text and talk. Social psychologists take the view that 'ideologies are above all discursive, instantiated within discursive actions ... Thus, the categories of ideology, together with shared stereotyping and commonplace social explanations, are framed in language' (Billig, 2002a, p. 184). Following Billig (1985, 1991), it is argued that prejudiced ideas can only be understood in their argumentative context. As Billig *et al.* (1988, p. 100) suggested,

> it is not difficult to view prejudice in a comparatively undilemmatic way, which assumes that the unprejudiced are liberal, healthy and egalitarian, whereas the prejudiced are the repositories of the very opposite values ... prejudice is not undilemmatically straightforward; there is a dialectic of prejudice.

Moreover, it is easy to assume that prejudice is just a matter of words, such as the verbal expression of commonplace stereotypes, while discrimination involves behaviour (the putting of prejudiced words into practice). Discrimination does not exist apart from words, utterances, expressions that enact discrimination in social settings. Our thinking is rhetorical, argumentative and dilemmatic. Thus, 'processes of everyday thinking can be processes of "ideology"' (Billig, 1991, p. 1).

Billig has highlighted the contrary nature of ideological themes, pointing to the ways in which people apply these in different contexts. Inconsistencies and contradictions point to the inherent ***dilemmatic*** quality of ideological thinking. As Wetherell and Potter (1992) have argued, 'the contradictory nature of ideological discourse permits considerable rhetorical flexibility and argumentative power' (p. 177). As Condor (1990) points out, people may not simply endorse or reject dominant views, but rather develop complex configurations of thought in which some dominant ideological elements find expression in conjunction with individual and group-based understandings (cf. also Augoustinos, 1998). Billig *et al.* (1988) distinguish between two meanings of ideology: the 'lived ideology' and the 'intellectual ideology'. The notion of 'lived ideology' refers to 'ideology as a society's way of life' (p. 27), including what passes for common sense within a society. 'Intellectual ideology' is defined as a 'system of political, religious or philosophical thinking and ... is very much the product of intellectuals and professional thinkers' (ibid.). The dilemmatic approach does not start with the assumption that there is an inner coherence to ideologies (Billig, 1991, 1992). Ideologies are fragmentary; they contain contrary themes. The ordinary person does not passively accept the (ideological) themes of intellectual ideology. As Billig (1991) has shown the ordinary person is a 'rhetorical being' who engages, and argues, with dilemmatic aspects of ideology. As Serge Moscovici has also written, 'social and intellectual activity is, after all, a rehearsal or recital, yet most socio-psychologists mistakenly treat it as if it were amnesic' (1984, p. 10).

Other social psychologists (cf. Wetherell, 1999, p. 403) call for a thorough exploration of 'ideology with a small i': 'why not focus, that is, more thoroughly on ideology with a small "i" (the mosaic of contradictory commonplaces and interpretative repertoires which organize everyday sense-making) rather than ideology with a capital "I" (coherent and global political systems of thought)?' A focus on ideology with a small 'i' can open ways for the exploration of specificity of ideological processes, embedded and reflecting very much of the social, political and ideological climate of specific socio-cultural contexts. According to this view, discourse is not inherently ideological, 'it becomes ideological in argument, debate and application' (Wetherell and Potter, 1992, p. 139). For discursive psychologists of racism, ideology is located in argument, in the intricacies of discourse about social issues such as prejudice (and what it means to be prejudiced), discrimination or inequality.

Discursive psychology, conversation and prejudice

Discursive psychology views opinions, beliefs and attitudes ('prejudiced' or otherwise) as resources that members can draw upon in talk, in order to accomplish contextual relevant rhetorical and social action (Wiggins and Potter, 2003). Discursive psychologists emphasize the primacy of social and discursive practices and, as a consequence, have focused on conversational interaction in interviews or natural settings, or documents of various kinds (Potter, 2012).

Discursive psychological analyses of prejudiced discourses focus on evaluative practices that are flexibly produced for particular occasions (Speer and Potter, 2000; Tileagă, 2005). Social psychologists concerned with explicit and implicit measures of prejudice have been reluctant to deal with actual conversational interaction, preferring to explore prejudiced atttitudes in experiments, questionnaires, or implicit measures.

Take, for example, the use of interviews in discourse research. In discursive psychology, interviews are used for identifying and exploring participants' interpretative and evaluative practices rather than as instruments for accessing a set of attitudes and beliefs (Potter and Hepburn, 2005). The subjectivities of both interviewer and interviewee are locally produced, sequentially, in and through talk (Rapley, 2001). Wetherell and Potter (1992) and Widdicombe and Wooffitt (1995), both extended discourse-based studies that work principally with interview material, illustrate some of the analytic possibilities they provide. Edwards (2003), exploring the use of interviews in analysing racial issues, suggests that interviews on controversial topics such as prejudice, discrimination, ethnic categorization or stereotyping are not easy to interpret. These kinds of interview often entail contradictory, ambiguous and ambivalent statements, and it is the task of analysis to disentangle the subtle choreography of direct, ambiguous or ambivalent prejudices, and how evaluations of prejudice (and what it means to be prejudiced) are produced in interaction to perform actions. Discursive psychologists treat members' talk as a topic of inquiry in its own right and their aim is not to theorize 'prejudice' per se, but to describe and explore the social meaning of prejudice for members of society, including orientations to norms against the expression of direct prejudice (Rowe and Goodman, 2014). Discursive psychologists examine the ways in which concerns with 'prejudice' inform social actors' reasoning; they explore how social actors describe, define and orient to prejudice as a matter of social relations between people, by drawing on the wider social context of intergroup relations (Tileagă, 2005, 2006, 2007). The aim is to draw attention to the various situated ways in which prejudice is identified, described, explained and made sense of in everyday or researcher-led encouters.

A number of discursive psychological studies of racism have highlighted the way in which concerns about being regarded as speaking from a prejudiced position are managed by constructing evaluations as mere factual descriptions, unmotivated by an inner psychology of ethnic or racial hatred (Edwards, 2003; Tileagă, 2005). For example, as Edwards (2003) shows, participants may inoculate themselves against the potential of their remarks being interpreted as prejudicial or biased by constructing their views as 'rationally arrived at'. Discursive psychologists have shown how denials of prejudice often appear together with 'practical', 'factual' reasons for furthering and preserving the status quo (Wetherell and Potter, 1992). They are interested in describing, accounting for, 'the precise manner by which people articulate a complex set of positions that blend egalitarian views with discriminatory ones' (Augoustinos and Every, 2007, p. 138).

Discursive psychologists do not try to see whether the speaker is 'really' prejudiced. Researcher-designed interviews or naturally occurring conversations, as sites of sociality, offer a fertile ground for researching public prejudices, without making any assumptions about the 'negativity' of statements, remarks and/or a putative 'faulty' psychology of individuals. For instance, conversation-analytic studies (Speer and Potter, 2000; Stokoe and Edwards, 2007) show how prejudice is sustained by routine conversational practices. Stokoe and Edwards (2007) and Stokoe (2009) show how members of society employ identity categories to talk about each other, and how social actions (such as blaming, accusing, discounting or diffusing responsibility, complaining, etc.) are actions done by using identity categories. Identity categories organize, and distill, complex cultural knowledge about appropriate, or expected, behaviours of others.

In their analysis of racial insults in neighbour complaints and police interrogations, Stokoe and Edwards (2007) show how racial insults are carefully constructed and reported. A common practice was to pair ethnic identity categories with an injurious word (e.g. 'gypsy twat' or 'Paki bastard'). Interestingly, as Stokoe and Edwards observe, talk about ethnicity and racism was, with regularity, formulated in 'reported speech' (that is, by voicing the words of another) and embedded in complaint sequences. Reported speech has been shown to be a powerful rhetorical resource to articulate to justify problematic accounts or views on race (Buttny, 1997). In social settings, racial abuse (racial insults), and responses to these, can take various forms. Stokoe and Edwards write about a continuum of responses 'from explicit second assessments done in ordinary talk, to minimal but affiliative responses in mediation calls, to an absence of response in police interviews' (2007, p. 367). Insults are not just a matter of tying identity categories and negative terms or stereotypes, but they also facilitate the construction of some people, and their behaviour, as 'complainable' (Schegloff, 2005).[1]

Studies of conversational sexism (e.g. Speer and Potter, 2000) show how social interactions facilitate the production and negotiation of prejudice *in situ*. Discursive analysis is not a tool for capturing the 'negativity' or 'irrationality' of prejudices, or for mapping 'a type of talk on to a type of person' (p. 564), but is rather a tool for making sense of how participants themselves produce and make sense of prejudice. The acceptability or the offensiveness of heterosexist remarks, Speer and Potter argue, is something attended to in interaction.

Studies that concentrate on the discursive analysis of semi-structured interviews on ethnic and racial issues (e.g. Tileagă, 2005; Verkuyten, 2001) highlight the (often downplayed) role of the interviewer in the production of prejudicial statements. In social interaction, it is people who occasion, reinforce or suppress the expression of prejudiced beliefs. The dialogic nature of conversations (whether naturally occurring or interview-based) 'allows us to recognize how the success, or otherwise, of a claim to non-prejudiced character ultimately depends upon its acceptance or rejection on the part of an audience' (Condor *et al.*, 2006, p. 458). Arguably, it does matter when and how prejudice is relevant or salient, and who gets to decide that it is; when and how words or actions are motivated by 'hate', 'contempt' or mere conjecture, and where they are not (Whitehead, 2009). In ordinary conversations and/or interviews various discursive practices (explicit or implicit assessments, explicit or minimal affiliative responses, repairs) show that prejudice is a subtle collaborative accomplishment and, more importantly, define the various (tolerant, ambivalent or extreme) trajectories of public prejudice.

It is, therefore, important to take into account how co-conversationalists orient to, respond to and position themselves regarding the social acceptability of what is being said. If prejudice is an interpretive concept, then researchers need to pay close attention to how it is interpreted, oriented to, monitored, 'policed' by members of society. Focusing exclusively on negative description of groups in conversation (through stereotyping, or other means of negative evaluation) without taking into account the idea that there is also a lot of ambiguity, allusion, indirectness in the expression of public prejudice, and that people themselves regulate the expression of prejudice, provides only a partial understanding of public prejudice.

However, one cannot understand the grounds of co-conversationalists' orientations to the social acceptability of prejudices without also taking into account that prejudiced talk is intricately woven with macro-level societal assumptions about what is acceptable, who is entitled to and worthy of equal treatment, and what are the bounds of rational and reasonable behaviour towards others.

The social acceptability of prejudices

Discourse analysis is a useful tool for analysing discourse (prejudiced or otherwise) by 'carving out a piece of the argumentative social fabric for closer examination' (Wetherell, 1998, p. 405). The argumentative social fabric that Wetherell alludes to comprises the extensive range of lay and elite assumptions, presuppositions, about the social inclusion and exclusion of people that each society uses as background. In everyday and researcher-led conversations, individuals (co-interactants) occasion, reinforce or fail to suppress prejudice (Condor *et al.*, 2006). As Condor argues,

> in the course of ongoing conversational interaction racially or ethnically prejudiced talk may also be used to perform a wide range of communicative functions: to amuse, to seize the floor, to exclude, to shock, to mark intimacy, to key informality, to display freedom from normative constraint or simply to pass the time.
>
> (2006, p. 15)

Conversation is the privileged medium of sociality, and indeed it would be odd if we did not take into account the various communicative functions of talk. Condor does not wish to suggest that audibly, recognizably prejudiced talk is innocuous but that, in conversation, it is not necessarily the expression of inner mental states. Prejudiced cognitions are distributed cognitions; that is, their expression is socio-communicatively shared with those people who share the same assumptions about the social acceptability/unacceptability of prejudices.

But one cannot truly understand the wider question, and implications, of the social acceptability of prejudices without moving beyond micro-social, face-to-face encounters.

At a broader, societal level, societal assumptions and repertoires about the social worth of people occasion, reinforce or sanction the active social imaginary that feeds into the social acceptability/unacceptability of prejudices, and the direct as well as indirect expression of prejudice against certain groups of people. The media is one of the principal channels through which societal assumptions are reproduced. Research studies that consider media representations of ethnic groups and racism (Erjavec, 2001; Lynn and Lea, 2003) point to thematic and form structures of news and media reports that work to legitimate and naturalize unequal treatment of people designated as different or unentitled to, or unworthy of, equal treatment. In the case of Romani people, one can see a continuum of representation, from hackneyed group caricatures that promote stereotypes in the service of shallow entertainment (see, for instance, the popularity of TV shows such as *Gypsy Brides*, *My Big Fat Gypsy Wedding*, etc.) to ambivalent, and sometimes questionable, portrayals of Roma individuals and communities afflicted by irremediable poverty and destitution.

The Internet encourages the expression of (extreme) views without the same level of policing, or suppression, as in ordinary conversations. For instance, blatant sexism is rife on Facebook and Twitter. Extreme views against Romani people (which can be found on the majority of run-of-the-mill newspaper discussion forums around Europe) arouse little suspicion from editors or little opposition from other ordinary users. The salience and weight of an operative social norm against prejudice in conversation is significantly diluted in online environments.

What is also increasingly clear is that there seems to be an emergent norm against making accusations of racism (Augoustinos and Every, 2007). As Goodman and Rowe (2014) show, when it comes to the Roma, accusations of racism on discussion forums are met with criticism, and a distinction is made between 'prejudice' and 'racism'. Blaming Roma (Gypsies) for their own predicament may be seen as prejudice, but not racism. Moreover, people accusing others of racism are perceived as closing off legitimate debate and curtailing freedom of speech (Goodman and Burke, 2010). However, generally, blaming Romani people for their own predicament is considered acceptable. The acceptability of blaming the victim seems to be tied to the idea that the Roma (Gypsies) are unlike any other group. Ordinary members of society, as well as elites, work on the assumption that the quality and nature of prejudice varies with the perceived worth of the target group. For instance, Tileagă (2006) has shown that middle-class prejudices against the Hungarian minority in Romania are qualitatively different from those against the Roma. Middle-class Romanian professionals differentiate very carefully between different types and intensities of prejudice. Whereas anti-Hungarian prejudices are underpinned by nationalistic undertones, anti-Roma prejudices are either deeply ambivalent, or extreme, in their eliminationist connotations. It is not uncommon for middle-class participants to exhibit some orientation to the problematic nature of negative portrayal of Gypsies, but would not necessarily call it 'racism', and would not necessarily directly challenge views that contend that Roma (Gypsies) are 'dirty', 'lazy', 'criminal', 'fail to integrate', etc. Tileagă noticed the presence and influence of a societal taboo against prejudice, but this was embraced only half-heartedly, and reluctantly, by otherwise law-abiding, reasonable individuals. *How* to talk about the Roma without being seen as prejudiced or racist was a live concern. However, unguarded prejudices spilled unrestrained in the conversations between interviewer and interviewee. There was a sense that, somehow, it was acceptable to talk about Romani people in a direct, unguarded way. The operative relevance of principles of equality, justice or fairness was drawn upon when middle-class Romanians were talking about the Hungarian minority, but the same principles were not applied when talking about Romani people.

Frequent comparisons between groups (Romanians, Hungarians and Roma) were a very common strategy used to portray the Roma as inadequate, unworthy of equal treatment. As other studies have shown, comparisons between ethnic minority groups are used to construct a specific and distinctive negative ethnic identity (see Verkuyten *et al.*, 1995). Instances where Roma are compared with the majority population as well as other ethnic minority groups revealed the persistence of unfavourable evaluations couched in the language of reasonableness and (irreversible and essential) cultural differences. Examples below, from semi-structured interviews with middle-class

Romanian professionals, are illustrative of this move. Interestingly, this can be found across the spectrum of views and support for progressive, tolerant or conservative, discriminatory politics and policies. Marc (Extract 5.1), a 51-year-old high school teacher, is a person who has previously expressed unwavering support for exclusionary right-wing policies, whereas Valeria (Extract 5.2), a 25-year-old primary school teacher, has expressed a more ambivalent position towards exclusionary right-wing policies. In contrast, Andrei (Extract 5.3), a 54-year-old accountant, has expressed his firm opposition to the exclusionary policies of Romanian right-wing politicians.

Extract 5.1

```
Chris  What is your view of the position, the social and economic status
       of national and ethnic minorities in the past and today? (.) The
       social, economic position (.) I am referring mostly to Hungarians,
       Romanies (.) Germans, less numbered now (0.5)
Marc   Their situation (.) talking about the main minorities, so the
       Hungarians (.) there is no difference, Hungarians, Germans,
       Serbs (.) in comparison with the Romanians (.) they are similar
       (.) they can fulfil themselves and can accomplish a social position
       (.) anyone of them (.) the Gypsies (.) however, in comparison to
       how they were (.) years ago, they've also risen on the social scale
       (.) some of them at a material level (.) but culturally, there is
       still something missing (.)
```

In Extract 5.1 Marc is answering a question about the 'status' of ethnic minority groups. The question of the interviewer is a rather complex one and, theoretically, not amenable to a simple answer. Marc picks up the implication of the interviewer's question – that there might be some discrete differences between ethnic groups. From the outset Marc is careful to distinguish between different *types* of minorities – on one hand, the 'main minorities' (l. 286), and, on the other hand, 'the Gypsies' (l. 290). Note the subtle use of the term 'the Gypsies' instead of the interviewer's 'Romanies'. As Leudar and Nekvapil (2000) argue, 'membership categories are prior resources for talking about people' (p. 492). In a carefully designed concessionary move (Antaki and Wetherell, 1999), Marc brings to the fore the trope of 'cultural' backwardness. Marc's category work is twofold. On one hand, he concedes that 'Gypsies' are comparable on some aspects ('at a material level'). On the other hand, at a more profound level, 'Gypsies' are found to be lacking what all the other groups *own*, or take for granted/share in common: 'culture'. Interestingly, this is presented as something that 'is still [...] missing' – an essential difference between groups. What Marc gives with his initial description of Gypsy material betterment he takes back by highlighting essential 'cultural' differences between groups.

Although having conceded a positive transformation, it can be argued that Marc's overall stance is one of criticism rather than sympathy. By making relevant, yet unspecified, 'cultural' differences, Romanies are relegated to a single, 'special' category differentiated in talk from a composite category of cultured, civilized others, which includes majority Romanians and other cohabiting ethnic groups. We can see how the issue of Romani status or worth is discussed with reference to a distinction between 'material' and 'cultural' status or worth. Whereas 'material' status is something that can be acquired, 'culture' is something intrinsic to the person and to the group to which the person belongs. Marc's use of the term 'culture' is slipping between the two meanings of 'culture', a particular meaning (of cultural differences), but also a universal meaning (of culture as civilization). It is the second (universal) meaning that Marc is drawing upon to pass a judgement on Romani moral standing in the world. The implicit (cultured, civilized, enlightened) standard of the 'main minorities' is accorded privileged status in the comparison (cf. Sampson, 1993).

In Extract 5.2 the interviewer addresses a question about the issue of extending the rights, and privileges, of the ethnic and national minorities.

Extract 5.2

```
Chris    Do you think that the rights (.) the privileges of national and
         ethnic minorities should be extended? (.)
Valeria  Their rights? (.) If they should be extended more? (1.8)
         I do::nt think so
         (0.2)
Chris    Think of the Hungarians, the Germans and the Gypsies (.) they
         are too (.)
Valeria  Well, this is the point (.) that (1.2) if (.) even from their
         point of view one can notice a (.) a desire to ameliorate the
         situation, then yes (.) okay (.) let's extend them (.) nobody
         has a problem with it, as long as this doesn't lead to
         (.) conflicts, for example, as there were then (.) So (.) I am
         talking for example now about the Gypsies, I am thinking that
         they practically do not have as many rights as (.) as the
         Germans, as the Hungarians (0.7) But (.) not being civilized,
         they don't know how to (.) to have pretences (.) to take
         advantage of this
         (0.5)
         yes, they don't even know how to take advantage (.) because they
         are complacent in that situation (.) being the way they are (.)
```

The list that the interviewer offers at line 365 seems to invite a comparison and also to imply that there might some kind of differences between the groups listed. Mentioning the Gypsies as the third element of the list seems to trigger an immediate reaction. After a short preface (ll. 367–371), Valeria reframes the issue of rights for the Gypsies as something that pertains to their 'culture' and 'way of being' (ll. 372–378). As Marc, Valeria is drawing upon the notion of Romani cultural backwardness, to put together a verbal portrait of Romani mentality.

The formulation ('being the way they are') at line 379 is telling in this context. One can read this as an extreme comment, an essentialist 'theoretical rationalization' (van Leeuwen and Wodak, 1999). It is not just the characteristics of Romanies that are essentialized, but also their ontological 'being' in the world. Valeria reduces them to the *essence* of their essence. This portrayal of Romanies excludes them from moral membership in the wider social and political community. It alters, transforms, their individual and collective worth in the eyes of their fellow human beings.

Both Marc and Valeria speak from the assumption that it is socially acceptable, and reasonable, to describe Romani people as essentially, culturally backward. A Romanian poll conducted in 2009 showed that whereas Romanians and Hungarians tended to be described in broadly similar terms ('thrifty', 'trustworthy', 'welcoming', 'intelligent'), Roma were described as 'lazy', 'thieves' and 'backward' (IMAS, 2009). Both Marc and Valeria draw on the available social repertoires about the social acceptability of prejudices against the Roma. Marc and Valeria speak from within the universal community of the 'civilized', the 'settled', the 'normal' and the 'reasonable', for whom it is acceptable to place Romani people beyond difference, and beyond a taken-for-granted civilized moral order.

In Extract 5.3, Andrei volunteers a response to a question about the existence of prejudices against the Hungarian minority. He draws on an explicit contrast with 'the gypsies' to substantiate the absence of prejudices against Hungarians. Andrei does not trade in stereotypical descriptions but offers instead a commentary on the (perceived) status and worth of Romanies (ll. 327–332).

Extract 5.3

Chris Do you think that Romanians are prejudiced against the Hungarians or not really?
Andrei No, no (0.4) I don't know (1.2) The ordinary Romanian, he has nothing against the Hungarian, with the gypsy (0.2) With the gypsies is more (.) Towards gypsies they have prejudices, because I told you, these ones don't work (.) The Hungarians have no problems, they are integrated in society (.) and where they work, it is obvious Hungarians are a hard working people=
Chris Hmm
Andrei =As I went through the county, I took a look at Valea lui Mihai, at Sacuieni, the land was laboured (.) Salard, so it was a work done with love, with (.) So, the Hungarians must be appreciated from this point of view=
Chris yeah
Andrei =they are a hard working people (.) While gypsies, for the gypsies there is a complete revulsion=
Chris mhm
(0.4)
Andrei =for the gypsies
(0.2)

Whereas Andrei's praising comments about the Hungarians allude to a shared assumption of similarity, Andrei's 'revulsion' statement about the Romanies is based on an assumption of *complete* and *extreme difference*. The Hungarians and the Romanies are not two sides of the same coin; the two groups are said not to share the same symbolic, moral space of worth. 'Revulsion' is the operative word, an umbrella-term, a description, for everything that is negative about the Romanies and need not be stated. In this extract, this description does not appear alone and it is the more insidious as it appears alongside positive descriptions of Hungarians and is upgraded by the use of an extreme case formulation ('complete revulsion').

This description dehumanizes the Roma and makes relevant a sense of Romanies as 'abject' (Kristeva, 1982), as matter 'out of place'. I consider separately the issue of dehumanization in the next chapter. Andrei does not claim to be personally revolted by the Romanies, but talks about 'revulsion' in general terms. There is a shift of footing from a story of personal involvement in the case of the Hungarian minority to an impersonal way of talking about 'revulsion' as far as the Romanies are concerned. Andrei describes revulsion as something pervasive and general, but not something necessarily associated with the feelings, wishes and motives of a particular individual. Rhetorically, Andrei addresses a universal, reasonable audience to which the idea, the notion, that Romany 'behaviour' is disgusting or repulsive is non-controversial. This is a claim for reasonableness based on the implicit idea that everyone would feel the same (that is, disgusted) about Romanies and their behaviour. As Marc and Valeria, Andrei alludes to the social acceptability of prejudices and negative evaluations of Romanies. He speaks on the assumption that it is socially acceptable, and reasonable, to describe Romani people as repulsive (especially when they are contrasted with other groups). Although Andrei is the kind of person that firmly opposes elite right-wing extremism, he does not express an alternative view nor does he qualify what he said. The consequences of such a position is that Romanies are denied moral worth and the status of moral subjects. Talk about revulsion, as well as cultural backwardness, include orientations to the moral standing, the moral worth of people. In these extracts, there is an asymmetry and inequality of rhetoric that gives more moral 'credit' and status to 'us' (Romanians) and other ethnic groups, but, at the same time, denies moral legitimacy and moral worth to the Roma.

What Graumann has called 'moral discrimination' (1998) is a notion relevant here. The evaluative judgements in these three extracts are not accidental, they are not made based on fortuitous criteria; they are made on *moral* grounds. These evaluative judgements are moral evaluations, moral judgements (Bar-Tal, 1989, 1990). Romanies are placed 'outside the boundaries of the commonly accepted groups' (Bar-Tal, 1989, p. 171). The issue of cultural backwardness and that of revulsion is presented as an incontrovertible issue of 'incommensurable identities' (Bhabha, 1992); on the one hand, 'us', the 'civilized', the 'normal' (Romanians, Hungarians, Germans – generally, 'European'), on the other hand, the Romanies, 'uncivilized', 'abnormal', 'deviant', 'disgusting'. Romanies are not only part of a different 'moral universe', but they *are* this different moral universe; a universe of extreme difference, transgressive, non-normative behaviour. As I will be showing in the next chapter, in this alternative moral universe it is not stereotypical negative descriptions that matter but certain, more complex descriptions of Roma as out of place, out of sync with what are seen as 'civilized' and 'decent' standards of behaviour.

Analysing discourse closely can help us think about societal repertoires around the social acceptability prejudices. Prejudiced talk contains explicit and implicit orientations to what counts as acceptable ways of talking about (certain) people. Making comparisons between groups is only one way to orient to the social acceptability of prejudices. Certain ways of talking about different, but outwardly similar, minorities implies that prejudices against other minorities like the Romanies are not only warranted, but also socially acceptable – arguably, the last acceptable prejudices. The conventional norm against prejudice of which Billig writes reflects the idea that the social acceptability of prejudices changes over time, and that individuals will ultimately internalize the moral demands of living together. Social psychologists, as well as historians, anthropologists or sociologists, point to historical shifts from acceptability to unacceptability of certain prejudices. For instance, in the United States, it has been found that students tend to report having only prejudices that are acceptable (Crandall *et al.* 2002). This is not surprising given that there is a norm against the expression of unwarranted prejudice. The 'prejudiced' are those who fail to observe, and internalize, this norm. These are the 'people who are behind the times, who fail to adapt easily to shifting standards of decency' (Crandall *et al.*, 2013, p. 63).

But what we are increasingly noticing is the contrary: it is the people 'of the times' who are prepared to alter, transform and limit the standards of decency! The social norm against prejudice only extends to prejudices construed as unwarranted prejudices. Moral exclusion prejudices (like prejudices against Roma) perpetuate and are resistant to criticism because they are presented as rational and warranted prejudices.

The issue of acceptability of prejudices is not that people conform to what they believe to be acceptable behaviour in their group(s). This view uncritically accepts an individual-differences view that claims to be able to distinguish between people on the basis of different intensities of norm-following behaviour, and defines prejudice as 'negative evaluation'. What discursive studies have shown is that the matter of acceptability of prejudices is more complex. Public prejudices are not just a matter of self-adaptation to (new) social norms but rather an issue of language, collective definition and the social meaning of prejudice at societal level (Tileagă, 2014).

Conventionally, it is believed that changing normative climates lead to changes in attitudes. People's motivation to suppress prejudice may be high or low, and/or may be linked with the prevailing social norms. Social norms against prejudice are perhaps more fluid than we allow. What Europe has witnessed from the first wave of admissions in 2004 to the most recent inclusion of Romania and Bulgaria into the European project is how citizens of Western liberal democracies (societies with strong norms against prejudice) are showing marked uneasiness in upholding the values of equal treatment and justice for all. Faced with (seemingly 'uncontrolled') movements of people, European citizens, and nation-states, rewrite the collective definitions of prejudice. They invent new rhetorical tropes and justifications for thinking about the 'new' immigrants, including the moral status of the Roma. They reinvent the rhetorical grounds for holding both prejudiced and tolerant attitudes.

Anti-Roma prejudices are one of the last acceptable contemporary European prejudices. As Allport would argue, they are part of a class of 'stubborn' prejudices. Anti-Roma prejudices tend to oscillate between visibility and invisibility, between suppression and extreme expression. 'Stubborn', historical prejudices reflect multiple forms of oppression or domination and are not satisfactorily explained by individual differences between people.

Anti-Roma prejudices are multiple and Romani people experience multiple forms of inequality, domination and degradation – gender, health, employment, housing, etc. These forms of inequality, domination and degradation are interlinked. Across the political spectrum views are aired that refuse dignity and a moral status in the world to the Roma. Rational, seemingly liberal positions (and not only extreme positions, as I have shown in Chapter 3) connect themselves, symbolically, to a history of Roma persecution.

To focus on the irrational or flawed psychology of individuals would be to miss the ideological weight of anti-Roma prejudices. Policing the expression or suppression of racism is not only present in the 'delicate choreography of everyday sociability' (Condor, 2006, p. 15) but also at the macro-social, societal level, in assumptions about the social acceptability of certain prejudices against certain people. Discourse analysis can offer a solid grounding for engaging with the complex societal nuances of racism. Discourse analysis can reveal how accounting for people's (Roma's) moral worth is tied to the range of operative social practices and societal principles that regulate the acceptability/unacceptability of expressions of prejudice and the ways of talking, repertoires, they produce and sustain.

Notes

1 What Schegloff calls the 'complainability of conduct' is a major part of understanding, and researching, prejudice as an everyday occurrence in conversation. This includes complaints about transgression and misconduct that have implications for the moral portrait of the transgressor. As I illustrate in the next chapter, complaints about transgression are routine ways by which one can construct people's behaviour, and their character, as incompatible, or antagonistic, to a 'civilized' moral order.

Chapter 6

Beyond stereotypes

Moral transgression and being 'out of place'

In the preceding chapter I indicated that comparisons between different ethnic minority groups are a resource for relegating Romani people to a position of extreme difference, and portraying them as people out of sync with civilized behaviour. Although I used examples from research with majority group members, what I described is not dissimilar to how Romani people are routinely presented in the media and, generally, in national and European public spheres: Roma are routinely portrayed and perceived as being unlike any other group, failing to integrate and failing to observe minimal standards of decency, due to the existence of incommensurable cultural differences. In the eyes of majorities, and other groups and communities, Romani people are not judged on an equal footing; they acquire special status and, as a consequence, merit special treatment.

In this chapter I extend the narrative from Chapter 5 and argue that, although the contemporary portrayal of Roma across Europe relies on stereotypical portrayals such as laziness, distaste for work, criminality, inferior mentality and so on, the source of discourses and practices that morally exclude them is a much broader moral and societal consensus of Roma as unworthy and undeserving of equal treatment, 'out of place' and transgressors of fundamental moral values. Like in Chapter 5 I use examples of majority-group members talking about the Roma, but also make reference to other contexts and settings.

The stereotypical image of the Roma depicts them as failing the various tests of 'worth' that societies impose on their citizens. When talking about Romani people, majority-group members attribute stereotypical traits to the Roma in not simply abstract but, rather, carefully, socially contextualized stereotypes. When contextualized, stereotypes become ways of (collectively) imagining the presence and worth of the Roma. Contextualized stereotypes also become ways of marking boundaries and evaluating the social distance between groups. Imagining the Roma as being beyond the bounds of what is reasonable in contemporary society, failures according to societies' motivational schemes, presupposes a moral discourse that presents them as unworthy, undeserving of equal treatment, and that excludes them from full citizenship. This imagining depends upon wider societal concerns with (1) the social (and moral) distance between groups, (2) moral evaluations of Romani behaviour in dispositional terms and (3) moral and spatial transgression. Only by understanding the reach, and function, of these wider societal concerns can one understand the depth and breadth of Romani marginality in Europe. In the remainder of this chapter I discuss these three aspects in turn.

From social to moral distance

Frequent comparisons between ethnic minority groups, of the kind presented in Chapter 5, reflect assumptions of what social psychologists and sociologists describe using the term 'social distance' (Bogardus, 1928; Triandis and Triandis, 1962). Unlike discourse analysis that proceeds by analysing stretches of talk, social distance measures conceive of prejudice as a concrete manifestation of dislike, mediated by the quality and willingness of social contacts, social relations and social interactions. Social distance measures represent prejudice as a concrete, contextualized phenomenon, with roots in everyday (spatial and symbolic) sociality.

Social distance measures on the Roma aim to capture a global evaluation of the group without reference to any specific stereotypical content. Social distance measures are used widely on research on the Roma on their own (Mărginean, 2001) or alongside other measures (Rughinis, 2012), and are included in reports to substantiate claims about the (continuous) social and moral exclusion of the Roma. For instance, in Romania, ethnic barometers show an increase of ethnic tolerance (e.g. Fleck and Rughinis, 2008). However, although Romani people tend to be accepted and included at the general level of the community ('living in the same country or town', 'learning in same classroom', 'working for the same company'), a symbolic fear of miscegenation persists – Romani people should not marry into Romanian families. More generally, they are described as people that 'are not to be trusted' (cf. IMAS, 2009). At the European level, a recent (special) Eurobarometer on 'Discrimination in the European Union' argues that 'overall, Europeans are very comfortable with the idea of having someone from a different ethnic origin than theirs as a neighbour' (European Commission, 2008, p. 6). Yet, when one inspects the data on Romani people, the average 'comfort' score drops significantly.[1] According to the Eurobarometer 'Discrimination in the EU in 2012', Europeans are more tolerant, more open-minded, 'increasingly accepting of diversity in the public sphere' (European Commission, 2012, p. 7). Yet, Romani people continue to have the lowest score on acceptance as a member of one's family (see also Fleck and Rughinis, 2008). Although Europeans are presented as more open-minded, more tolerant, their everyday behaviours and actions towards Romani people show marked moral ambivalence and moral uneasiness.

Although social distance measures can give us some information on the gradation of explicit attitudes and on the explicit positioning of other groups in the landscape of social relations, it is the power of symbolism of social relations with a certain category of people that informs the intensity and direction of prejudiced attitudes. When one analyses talk one starts to appreciate the rhetorical complexity of prejudiced attitudes; one also starts to appreciate that issues of social distance and contact cannot be apprehended without taking seriously the symbolic, or dilemmatic, aspects that underpin descriptions of the moral distance between Romani people and other groups.

As I showed in Chapter 5, operative and prevailing norms of moral distance that portray Romani people as out of sync with civilized behaviour can be seen across the attitudinal spectrum. Social distance turns into moral distance, social exclusion turns into moral exclusion, when people's individual and community worth and dignity are not fully recognized, when it is altered or transformed without possibility of retort and when it is seen as deficient, incomplete, out of place.

Moral evaluations and disposition

A striking feature of descriptions of Roma behaviour, of their way of being in the world, is implicit or explicit constructions of what sort of people Roma *are*. Interestingly, what explains Roma's behaviour is not motive or stake, but a certain ***psychological disposition*** to behave in a way that is contrary to the values of the 'settled' and 'civilized'. In this section I explore what discursive psychologists call 'disposition talk' (Edwards, 2003; Tileagă, 2007) as a resource for blaming Romani people for their own predicament and delegitimizing their ways of being in the world. Disposition formulations are

> ways in which whatever one is saying about the world is presented as fixed in that world, and rationally inferred from it, rather than residing in the speaker's ways of seeing.
>
> (Edwards, 2003, p. 42)

Extracts 6.1 and 6.2 are examples of such talk.

Extract 6.1 (a discussion about the causes of interethnic conflict)

Chris	To what extent do you think Romanies are to blame for these conflicts and violences?
Sandra	Cos' they don't (.) cos' they don't like to work (.) they <u>don't</u> like to work (.) They (.) Th[ey are not happy with-]
Chris	[How would you characte]rize them?
Sandra	Inadaptable (.) these ones are inadaptable (.) they cannot integrate in (.) in fact, even in the other countries (.) have their gypsies adapted? (.) No (.) Only that, it is the Romanians gypsies that Europe talks about, you have just these ones (.) it is only our gypsies that are the biggest thieves and bandits (.) But Romanians have tried to integrate them, we made them schools (.) they have TV shows in the gypsy (.) language (.) I have worked at a gypsy school (.) I use to bring them (.) I took care of them, every week, on Monday they used to come and after that, they didn't come all week (.) They cannot integrate, they like the life they are living (.)

Extract 6.2

Chris How would you characterize them if you were to draw a psycho-behavioural portrait of the Romanies, how would you characterize them (1.2)
Marc Less hardworking (.) less thrifty (.) they think less for the future (3.5) All this is linked with (.) education (.) so there is no preoccupation for education (.) and for their children (.)
I don't know (.)

In both extracts Romanies are presented as lacking something that is considered very important in the eyes of the dominant group. They are described as not sharing pivotal democratic and societal values: the values of work, education and integration in society. In both extracts the interviewer invites quite an explicit description of the Roma. Notice how the answers mobilize specific dispositional formulations: 'they don't like to work', 'they like the life they are living' (Extract 6.1), 'less hardworking, less thrifty', 'there is no preoccupation for education' (Extract 6.2), which are provided as rational and reasonable descriptions of what Roma generally *do*, and how they generally *are*. Dispositional formulations permit the expression of socially shared, acceptable and recognizable stereotypes about Romani people. These stereotypes are not neutral descriptions; they are moral descriptions, descriptions of Romanies' moral character (cf. Edwards, 1997). Dispositional formulations intimate that any difficulties that the Roma might encounter are of their own making. The extreme description 'inadaptable' (Extract 6.1, l. 387) implies not just difficulty in fitting, but the *impossibility* of fitting. The implication is that the reasons for this impossibility of fitting are very much part of the Roma character and way of being. Adaptation and integration stand as absolute conditions, which Roma have to fulfil in order to rightfully enjoy the benefits of society. Presenting people as inadaptable implies an accusation. The implication of the peremptory assertion at lines 396–397 (Extract 6.1) (which follows an apocryphal story of 'good will') is that, ultimately, integration means adopting 'our' way of life. 'Our' way of life is not in need of justification, for it is the source of legitimation. The most powerful expectation, that of making 'them' (Roma) be a bit more like 'us', is embedded in talk about Roma character and values.

Discourses of moral exclusion need not make explicit claims to 'nature' or biological differences; they can instead be based on a discourse of cultural differences and cultural propensities. What some discourse researchers have called 'culture as mentality' (Verkuyten, 1997) or 'culture as lifestyle' (Augoustinos *et al.*, 1999) is used to account for behaviours that deviate from normative cultural expectations. Disposition formulations are a way of 'fixing' cultural differences and propensities in the moral character of Roma. Disposition formulations are also ways in which one can construct a contrast between Roma backwardness and normative societal values and assumptions about integration, work, etc. Dispositional formulations are the building blocks of a discursive 'lay ontology' (Durrheim and Dixon, 2000) that naturalizes the moral character of Roma. Any stereotypical predicates attached to the category 'Roma' (Roma 'criminality', Roma 'inadaptability', etc.) are thus explainable with reference to the moral character of the Roma. In the context of majority-group accounting, as Wetherell and Potter suggest, 'culture discourse ... becomes a naturally occurring difference, a simple fact of life, and a self-sufficient form of explanation' (1992, p. 137).

When politicians talk about the Roma they are also alluding to cultural differences and present these as normative dimensions of conduct. When David Blunkett recently warned of tensions between residents of Page Hall in Sheffield and Slovakian Roma he argued that: 'We have got to change the behaviour and the culture of the incoming community, the Roma community, because there's going to be an explosion otherwise. We all know that.' The Slovakian Roma's 'way of being' is perceived as a problem. 'We all know that' is an explicit reference to a normative moral order, which generates its inadaptable, uncivilized antithesis. This normative moral order is not just the national moral order, but a universal moral order. The 'we' in 'we all know that' indexes the universal rationality and reasonableness of right-thinking and law-abiding citizens. Blunkett alludes to the problematic 'behaviour' and 'culture' of the incoming Roma as something that is recognizable, something expected, without, nonetheless, naming or identifying a specific issue. Talking about Roma in general terms has the effect of portraying them as typically morally transgressive social actors. Although no actual story of impropriety or misconduct is told, impropriety and misconduct are anticipated on the basis of a putative uncivilized moral character of Romanies.

Spatial and moral transgression

In everyday conversations about Romanies it is common for apocryphal stories of impropriety, misconduct, to be told. Apocryphal stories of impropriety, misconduct, are resources used by speakers and writers to paint the moral character of Roma and present them as a certain type of offensive, reprehensible and expendable people. In this section I show how descriptions of spatial transgression embedded in stories of impropriety, misconduct, are doing 'moral work' (Drew, 1998).

Extract 6.3

```
                 (...)
427   Sandra     they have received accommodation in a block of flats (.) well,
428              after they received it (.) they had the block brand new (.) at
429              (.) after a maximum of two months, the block was looking as if
430              it had been bombed (.) without windows, without doors (.) dirty
431              on the stairs (.) I have (.) I have no words (.)
```

Extract 6.4

```
        [...]
Carla   >they don't own land to cultivate, to farm< and when they were
        offered a place to stay or something (.) I saw it on televi[sion]
Chris                                                            [uh h]uh
Carla   that they've put their horses in (.) so (.) >even if there were
        flats< (.) where they managed to or (0.4) So (0.4) even them,
        what they receive, they ruin (.) so, they don't (0.8)° they don't
        respect, that's the thing° (.)
Chris   Hmm
        (1.2)
```

Descriptions of people, activities and state of affairs are not simply reports on the world. They are accountable discursive phenomena through which we recognizably display an action's (im)propriety or (in)appropriateness, and they provide 'a basis for evaluating the "rightness" or "wrongness" of whatever is being reported' (Drew, 1998, p. 295). Sandra's story in Extract 6.3 and Carla's in Extract 6.4 are typical examples of descriptions of transgression that are morally implicative; that is, they open up inferences as to the moral character, profile, of the transgressor. Sandra's moral indignation ('I have (.) I have no words', l. 431) contains an implicit condemnatory dimension. As Drew (1998) suggests, 'accounts produced in the context of talk in which moral work is quite overt and explicit appear to be generally condemnatory; that is they are associated with complaints about the behaviours of others (in "reconstructed" versions of their behaviour)' (p. 296).

The two stories (Extract 6.3, ll. 427–431 and Extract 6.4, ll. 87–90) are explicit formulations of (extreme) spatial transgression. In both stories Romanies are the grammatically active agents and are presented exclusively as members of the ethnic group and not as individuals. As Erjavec (2001) suggested, 'if they are denied individual images, they are also denied the opportunity to escape the habitual portrayal of the ethnic group resting on prejudices and stereotypes' (pp. 714–715).

Both Sandra and Carla are construing Roma conduct as intentional and deliberate to make manifest the transgression of normative standards of propriety and, hence, warrant their sense of moral indignation. Whereas Sandra uses a first-person assessment to express a sense of grievance ('I have no words', l. 431), Carla uses a generalized description ('°they don't respect, that's the thing°', ll. 89–90) that places the onus on the Romanies. Both stories portray Romanies as transgressive, as not obeying minimal rules of conduct, lacking respect for property and for 'our' (and a general) spatial and moral order. The vivid description of spatial transgression, with an implicit orientation to intentional and deliberate conduct, portrays not only behaviour but also people as offensive and reprehensible. Roma themselves are construed as offensive and reprehensible.

At the same time, the Roma get 'morally constituted' (Jayyusi, 1993) as being 'out of place'. The references to 'dirt' associated with the behaviour of Roma (see also Extract 6.5) enforce the idea of Roma as offensive and expendable.

Extract 6.5

```
        (...)
Sandra  I have brought them a sack of nice (.) clothes (.) they were
        walking in rags (.)
Chris   >Right<
Sandra  I have given them nice clothes, I have brought them a bag of food,
        cos' they were eating from the garbage (.) just to see the next
        say (.) the nice clothes that I've given to them to wear, to get
        changed (.) if I stayed with them they've changed clothes (.) if
        not (.) they've thrown them into the garbage container (.) well,
        I don't really know what to say (.) why do they behave like this?
        It means that they like living in dirt (.) in
        dirt (.)
        (...)
        there is (.) there is something (.) they don't like (.) that's
        why people say that the gypsies are koszos
```

In Extract 6.5, Sandra explains the inappropriate response to her magnanimous act by using an extreme dispositional formulation ('they like living in dirt', l. 420). She uses a disposition formulation (notice the emphasized 'like') as a way of saying that whatever she is claiming about Romanies is a characteristic of their disposition towards the world. The ascription of an inner disposition is a powerful rhetorical tool in the work of essentializing the attributed stereotypical traits of Roma. She expresses indignation by painting an abhorrent moral character trait of the Roma. The reference to 'living in dirt' is an explicit sign of a moral discourse that implicitly draws attention to the transgression of a moral boundary.

Sandra's discourse echoes the commonly held conception that people, like the Roma, who are perceived as transgressing moral (and spatial) boundaries are typically classified as 'matter out of place' (Sibley, 1994, 1995). Note the shift from talking about 'living in dirt' to ascribing an essential moral quality to the Roma through the use of 'koszos' (l. 424).[2] The implication of this shift is that 'dirt', 'filth' is not only something that Romanies 'like living in', it is also something that is essentially part of their being, it is *what they are*.[3] It is not just the characteristics of Roma that are essentialized, but also their ontological 'being in the world'. They are reduced to the *essence* of their essence.

It is implied that Roma do the things they do *because that is the way they are*. As Kristeva has argued, 'filth is not a quality in itself, but it applies only to what relates to a boundary and, more particularly, represents the object jettisoned out of that boundary, its other side, a margin' (1982, p. 69). This constructs Roma as 'somehow less than human' (Billig, 2002a, p. 185), as abject, as horrible by the standards of 'civilized' society (note also the presentation of this as knowledge-in-common, as something of a commonplace). There is an implicit allusion to the idea that they are a 'threat' to order, to cleanliness.

What is interesting about this type of talk is that it comes from people who, in other contexts, express strong views against the exclusionary values of right-wing extremism. General declarations of reasonableness, sympathy and expressions of tolerance are turned into specific accounts of impropriety that portray the Roma as failures on the motivational schemes of society. An example is offered in Extract 6.6, where Mircea is answering a question about Romanian prejudices against the Roma.

Extract 6.6

Chris Do you think that Romanians are prejudiced against the Romanies or not really?

Mircea They are (.) So, Romanians are prejudiced against Romanies. So they think that (.) they think that they are (.) So, they are thieves, they are so (.) And this happens also because of us, to a large extent, cos' we fixed them a label for a long time, but also because of them, because they don't (.) they also don't try (.) especially because they have all sorts of organizations, they are represented in Parliament and (.) and at a local level they have all sorts of organizations, support groups (.) and they don't try to raise themselves, so no (.) so, they don't want to surpass their own condition. So they say, listen, we are (.) poor, we are as we are, we have many kids, we don't use soap because it's expensive, we don't do that because of this then they determine, right (.) a sort of momentary revuls[ion]=

Chris [hmm]

Mircea =And when you see that he is a gypsy you cross to the other side even if maybe he's a poor man, as there are Romanians who are unwashed, there are also Hungarians who are unwashed (mm) But with them, with them is the first- also because of their clothes, which attracts the attention, you cannot help noticing a gypsy woman, and their way of speaking,so in general they have a way of speaking, they speak very loud so they can get noticed as being there, in order to automatically, to awaken revulsion so you would leave. so (.) them too (.) we also have to help them and they have to help themselves

Mircea's opening even-handedness (ll. 243–246) gives way to expressing more direct criticism of Roma's 'way of being': 'they also don't try' (l. 247), 'they don't try to raise themselves' (l. 251) or 'they don't want to surpass their own condition' (ll. 251–252). Note the shift from 'trying' (to raise themselves) to 'not wanting' (to surpass their own condition). As in previous examples, Romany 'character' and behaviour is invoked in order to make a case not only for what Romanies *do*, but also for what Romanies *are*. There is an oblique reference to dirtiness ('we don't use soap because it's expensive', ll. 253–254) together with direct references to the emotional and physical effect of their presence: 'a sort of momentary revulsion' (l. 255), 'revulsion' (l. 264). The extreme term 'revulsion' is used to describe their way of being (ll. 252–255), their appearance ('their clothes', l. 260) and 'way of speaking' (l. 262). This is not an avowal of being personally revolted by the Roma, but rather an account that warrants the reasonableness of being revolted.

Revulsion is the expression of the detestable, of the aloof, of the horrible, and is usually symbolically tied to the insidious register of impurity, uncleanness and pollution. It is common for reasonableness, sympathy and tolerance to mingle with constructions that present the Roma as 'abject' (Kristeva, 1982). The emotional correlate of the abject is disgust, rejection, condescension and withdrawal of contact. The use of extreme terms such as 'revulsion' embedded in seemingly tolerant and reasonable discourse are means of prescribing an ideological position for Roma, one that places them beyond the 'reasonable' bounds of society.

The public and media spheres are replete with apocryphal stories of transgression and misconduct. These stories portray Roma as *transgressive*, as not obeying minimal rules of conduct and as lacking respect for property and for 'our' (and a universal) spatial and moral order.

The contemporary conversations about the moral status that should be assigned to the Roma 'evoke discursive history' (Wetherell, 2001, p. 389), historical tropes of Roma's inadequacy, inadaptability, and current but also past social relations. Vladimir Meciar, former Prime Minister of Slovakia, was reported to have said that '[Roma] are antisocial, mentally backward, inassimilable and socially unacceptable'. The mayor of the Romanian town Baia Mare, Catalin Chereches, considered as an abuse the request by the National Council for Combating Discrimination to take down a wall that separated the local Roma community from an access route into town. The voice of everyday folk, councillors, mayors and prime ministers is the voice of the 'dispossessed' (Billig, 1978, p. 296), an anguished and rather angered voice that points to the fact that the moral order has been turned upside down and as a result 'we' (the community of the 'settled' and 'civilized') have to suffer the consequences.

Examples of behaviour (or outcomes of behaviour) that it is seen as violating social and moral conventions delegitimizes and dehumanizes the Roma and places them beyond what is perceived as acceptable, normative, appropriate. Romanies are the embodiment of what Kristeva has called 'uncanny strangeness' (1991, p. 182). They are portrayed as unruly, as abject, as a problem that can never be completely solved. Talking about them engenders uncomfortable uneasiness in relation to a 'foreign body' (Kristeva, 1982). In the next chapter I explore in more detail the particularities of such delegitimizing and dehumanizing talk.

Marginality and territorial indignity

Abjection is caused by anything that 'disturbs identity, system, order … does not respect borders, positions, rules' (Kristeva, 1982, p. 4). With extraordinary regularity, the Roma are described as an unruly body: they disturb the civilized system and order, they break rules and transgress boundaries. Everyday and media discourses do not just churn out stereotypes but offer grounds for the reasonableness of abjection. It does not matter whether you support or oppose right-wing policies or the exclusionary policies of the state, when it comes to talking about the Roma there is an emerging consensus that the Roma are unlike any other group. Moreover, there seems to be a difficulty with designating a place for the Roma; they are perpetually described as 'out of place', as not fitting a conventional (national and transnational) ideology of civilized and normative conduct.

When talking about different others we are also talking about ourselves, our community of beliefs, our values, etc., that we take for granted. As Dixon (2001) argues, 'the process of common identification may often entail the development of a more inclusive sense of *where we are* (and who belongs there with us)' (pp. 598–599, emphasis in original). A common trope of Roma moral exclusion in Europe is based on a collective imagining of Roma as unlike 'us', and not belonging here with 'us'. Implied or explicit descriptions of the abnormality, aloofness, of Roma are based on a 'banal' contemporary ideological common sense of a 'settled', established, fixed and unchangeable moral order. A set of normative principles is used to legislate against particular norms and principles held by Romanies themselves.

In Chapter 1 I argued that the Roma in Europe represent the return of the unruly collective – a collective that embodies *partial society*, whose rules, norms, behaviours do not square with the existing 'cultural schemes' of European liberal democracies. The national and European collective creed of liberal democracy embodies a cultural *totality* intolerant to anything partial, independent, alternative (Boltanski, 2011, p. 154). Solidarity, sympathy, protection under the law extend only to those who signify or are willing to conform to cultural totality. In the eyes of everyday folk, legislators and policy-makers, Romanies embody partial society. This leads to the expression of attitudes that mingle sympathy with deep ambivalence towards the Roma.

This deep ambivalence has a striking spatial character. For instance, even people who accept that evictions or displacements are a bad, immoral thing would nonetheless contend, like Jacques Delors did recently, that 'the Roma cannot go just anywhere' (Delors, 2011). These voices that claim that the Roma cannot go just anywhere are rational, reasonable, liberal voices. These are the voices that represent the universal community of the 'civilized', the 'settled', the 'normal' and the 'reasonable'. Liberal, reasonable individuals and communities are careful not to deny humanity to Romanies but, paradoxically, highlight them as the 'wrong sort' of human beings. As Rorty has cogently put it, 'the force of "us" is, typically, contrastive in the sense that it contrasts with a "they" which is also made up of human beings – the wrong sort of human beings' (1989, p. 190).

A group can be in the 'wrong' place if the stereotype locates it elsewhere (cf. Sibley, 1995). The stereotype locates Romanies on the margins, as nomads, as perpetual 'strangers'. As the Jews before them (until the nineteenth century at least), the Roma are eternal strangers in anybody's land. In an enlarged Europe, there seems to be a problem with the designation of a proper place for Romanies. Liberal democracies are intolerant of 'the non-national void' (Bauman, 1989, p. 53), of anything that moves unhindered and does not respect boundaries. In an enlarged Europe, liberal democracies' contact with (immigrant) Romanies exacerbates collective anxiety about supposed impropriety, space and place transgressions, etc. The 'popular diagnosis' (Becker, 1963) of their moral deviance does not treat them on an equal footing, does not assign them equal worth, but rather delegitimizes their conduct and way of being in the world, presenting them as violators of pivotal normative requirements. Romanies are unlike any other immigrants; they are routinely denied the status of 'moral' subjects, and are positioned in the realm of the aloof, detestable 'horror' (Jahoda, 1999).

Mobility, freedom of movement and the 'new nomadism' of the 'new', enlarged, Europe are not theoretical abstractions but facts of life. The uneasiness triggered by their particular manifestations, especially in relation to unwanted 'newcomers', is not so much a reflection of antipathy as of unwanted, repulsive, destitution. To the great majority of Europeans the presence of Romanies, the wretched face of European freedom of movement, creates marked moral uneasiness. For mayors, councillors, national and European elites, this moral uneasiness about people turns into moral uneasiness about public places and spaces. The increased presence and visibility of immigrant Roma in Europe's urban areas and town centres has generated a variety of reactions, debates and calls for action. The moral status assigned to the Roma is that of 'nomads', 'place invaders' (Kabachnik, 2010b). Roma mobility and/or attachment to place is not considered on an equal footing with that of the 'settled'. As Kabachnik argues, 'by failing to take place seriously, or by only using a very location-bound and traditional view of place, many writers reproduce centuries-old stereotypes about Roma and nomads being placeless wanderers and thus vastly different and inferior' (2010a, p. 205).

Urban areas, town centres and fields are spaces that are seen as being in need of protection against what is perceived or construed as unruly or antisocial behaviour. For example, recently, councils in England (Westminster, Birmingham, Nottingham, Southampton and Slough) demanded powers that would allow them to arrest people engaged in what they see as 'aggressive begging'. The need for more local powers is justified in terms of 'an overly burdensome process together with an increasingly pressurised judicial system and the existence of legal "grey areas" [that] have meant that antisocial individuals and groups have been able to slip through the net, causing havoc in urban areas'.[4] Arrest and, in extreme cases, forced eviction are means through which Roma's worth is being modified; they are 'stamps of dishonour' (Wacquant, 2008) that can lead to acute feelings of indignity. The European record of

Roma evictions is the most shameful in the continent's history. For instance, a recent report by the European Roma Rights Centre offers the following statistics for just one country, France: 'French authorities forcibly evicted more than 21.537 Romani migrants in 2013, more than double the total for 2012. Law enforcement officers carried out 165 evictions affecting almost 19.380 people. There were 22 evictions due to fire, affecting 2.157 Roma' (ERRC, 2014). The French authorities' actions resonate with Delors' phrase: 'the Roma cannot go just anywhere.' Evictions and forced removals are justified on grounds other than ethnicity and/or nationality: health and safety, or the risk they pose to the locality. Elsewhere too, in Greece, Italy or Romania, 'Roma continue to be targeted with forced evictions and resettled to isolated and segregated housing' (Amnesty International, 2014, p. 28). People who are denied freedom of movement and settlement are denied dignity. Forced evictions, removals and resettlements enact moral exclusion in plain view. Whereas immigrants are 'generally thought of as voluntary members of plural societies' (Berry, 2006, p. 30), Roma's aspirations to mobility, freedom of movement and desire for transience are construed as anomalous. Full protection under EU law is, according to a recent report by Amnesty International, 'a promise yet to be fulfilled' (Amnesty International, 2014, p. 28).

Violence against the Roma is not a thing of the past. Amnesty International has documented more than 120 extreme violent attacks in countries such as Hungary, the Czech Republic, Slovakia and Bulgaria between 2008 and 2012 (cf. Amnesty International, 2013). This violence takes place in societies that allow Romani people to become visible targets of violence with restricted ability to defend themselves. This is violence that, arguably, reflects a 'broad moral code about violence' (Jackman, 2001) that presents it as acceptable. The social definition of violence against Romani people stems from broader societal moral codes and arrangements that do not give it the same moral and legal weight as other forms of violence against people, and give it 'the appearance of blameless inevitability' (ibid., p. 463).

Individual violence against Romani people plays a central role in the maintenance of unequal and dominant social relations. Organizationally or state-mandated violence can take no less direct or extreme forms – evictions, confinement, isolation, etc., as 'routine strategies of control' that transform the legitimacy and social meaning of violence. Organizationally mandated violence (such as that commissioned by local councils) is strategic violence that disguises its primary aim – that of dislocating and demeaning people. Organizationally mandated violence is not perceived as socially deviant (or illegal) but rather popularly supported and delivered in the name of the common good. Organizationally mandated violence is mobilized to uproot what it sees and construes as morally deviant, transgressive behaviours.

Amongst the indignities that the Roma experience, what Wacquant (2008) has called 'territorial indignity' is perhaps one of the most significant. Removal and eviction are only one aspect of altering Roma's worth. Separation, isolation and confinement of some Roma in slums, ghettos and 'widely despised zones of relegation' (p. 272) are a product of state-ratified, liberal democratic policies. Slums, on the outskirts of European towns and cities, are spaces of extreme socio-spatial marginality (Vincze, 2013) where a 'taint of place' (Wacquant, 2008) is 'superimposed on the already existing stigmata traditionally associated with poverty and ethnic origin' (ibid., p. 238). As Wacquant argues, slums and ghettos are social mechanisms of ethnic and racial *confinement*, 'aimed at enclosing a stigmatized category in a reserved physical and social space that will prevent it from mixing with others and thus risk "tainting" them' (ibid., p. 153). The symbolic fear of contamination, pollution, keeps people like the Roma in their place, in dehumanized and dehumanizing locales such as urban landfills.[5] Even those who profess the highest degree of tolerance towards minorities consider the confinement of Romanies as a necessary evil. The main premise of perpetuating separation, isolation and confinement is that the *modus existendi* of Romanies is the antithesis of a possible *modus coexistendi*. This works to prescribe an ideological position for Romanies, one that places them beyond the 'reasonable' bounds of society, humiliates and degrades them.

The vagaries of indignity

Roma in Europe face a three-pronged attack on their worth and dignity as human beings. First, from the European far right, for whom a Europe of values is a sovereign Europe of citizens. The recent chant of supporters of the Front National in France for the 2014 European elections, 'On est chez nous!' ('We are in our own home!'), encapsulates a desire for a Europe of 'free and sovereign nations', for a 'Europe of peoples'. The chant resonates with UKIP supporters in Britain or with supporters of the Danish People's Party in Denmark. It encapsulates a desire to exclude others that are not seen to belong 'here', in our space, with 'us' (Dixon and Durrheim, 2000). The French chant relies on a seemingly 'banal' contemporary ideological common sense of a 'settled', established, fixed and unchangeable moral order of 'nations' (Billig, 1995). The chant is the voice of the 'dispossessed' (Billig, 1978, p. 296), an anguished (and angered) voice that points to the fact that the 'normal' moral order of sovereign states has been turned upside down by the European project. According to this view, a cosmopolitan Europe is a mistake that needs to be rectified as soon as possible, by whatever means. Roma are the expression of unwanted, wretched poverty and destitution in a New Europe. Moreover, according to Alexis Tsipras (leader of Syriza in Greece), this New Europe 'is repulsive and dangerous and needs to change'. Tsipras's New Europe is a world turned upside down, made of repulsive and dangerous people.

Second, Roma face attacks on their dignity from seemingly tolerant people (mostly middle-class professionals) – similarly angered and disenfranchised voices – who, whilst presenting an individual image of tolerance, express veiled, and sometimes direct, hostility by using collective tropes, imagery, symbolism, with deeply degrading and humiliating consequences. It is perhaps no accident, and no surprise, that the tropes of 'revulsion' and 'danger' feature so prominently in the discourse of the right wing. Yet, interestingly, they also feature in the discourses of sympathetic and seemingly tolerant people. The idea of extending the values that the majority group takes for granted (freedom of movement, freedom of settlement, etc.) to Romanies can lead to marked discomfort, uneasiness and anxiety, even for individuals, groups or communities that profess tolerance as a matter of course.

And finally, Roma face attacks on their dignity from European neoliberalism that values control, social order and the market economy more than it values human life. Instead of being 'embraced for being tenacious, resourceful and adaptable, and for maintaining cultural traditions that value social fluidity and cross-nation unity; all values that lie at the heart of the European ideal', Roma 'are seen as a systemic irritant to power and the status quo' (Baker, 2012). Being mindful of the language and imagery/symbolism we take for granted, or becoming more aware of individual latent biases, is only a first step towards standing up to the perpetuation of Roma's moral exclusion. Individual introspection might be a necessary first step but in the real world of nations, borders, movement of people, etc., understanding how society operates as a mechanism of control and moral exclusion is perhaps even more important.

Paradoxically, European societies are unsure where they stand on assigning a moral status to the Roma. The uncertainty shown by European societies reflects a collective uncertainty at the heart of European societies – it is a sort of uncanny uncertainty about the Roma's worth as people, about their rightful place in the social and motivational structures/schemes of European societies. European uncertainty creates and perpetuates many situations 'in which the scope of justice undergoes change' (Opotow, 2011, p. 207). Changing the scope of justice makes people who are not inside, or included in it, particularly vulnerable to moral exclusion, on a continuum from subtle to extreme moral exclusion.

This collective uncertainty goes deeper, and wider, to the fundamental liberal values of the European (inclusionary and progressive) project: freedom of movement, freedom of settlement, social justice for all, etc. The idea of extending these values unconditionally to Others provokes notable discomfort even amongst the most tolerant sections of European societies. The most common objections are that it is not practical, that nations should have the right to sovereign decisions, etc. These values are instead used to define the rights and worth of citizens against the rights and worth of Others.

Simply signing up for tolerance and/or respect for diversity is, arguably, not enough. Most liberal democratic societies do not want to be perceived as harbouring immoral state policies that disregard the value of human life, but actual practice points to the contrary. Collective images of respectability and civility stand in stark contrast with actual practices of dislocating, removing or confining people. Contemporary Europe imagines itself as a cosmopolitan, tolerant, values-based and values-driven community – but the crude reality of the moral exclusion of Roma within and from society tells a different story. There is one pivotal European (and universal) value – the right to life – that we seem to take for granted, but fail to extend it to Romani people. Under European law everyone should be entitled to protection against bodily harm and annihilation, extreme humiliation, forced removal, relocation or confinement. In this climate, the Roma themselves are unsure who they can turn to for help and protection.

Europe demands of its citizens to show enlightened tolerance, without first engaging in genuine introspection into its own practices of keeping others out of the scope of justice. This tolerant and cosmopolitan image of progressive Europe is shattered by the numerous examples of harsh, unfair and uncalled-for treatment of Romanies both in their home countries and abroad. Europe persists in professing its communal and community values for all, whilst at the same time perpetuating and enacting morally exclusionary policies that limit the freedom and freedoms of Romanies. The source of discourses and practices that morally exclude Romanies is steeped in a broader moral and societal consensus around Roma's unworthiness and moral transgression of fundamental liberal values.

Notes

1 As the authors of the 2008 Eurobarometer on discrimination argue: 'around a quarter (24%) of Europeans would feel uncomfortable having a Roma neighbour: a striking difference to the level of comfort with a person from a different ethnic origin in general (where only 6% would feel uncomfortable)' (European Commission, 2008, p. 8).

2 The word that Sandra uses to describe the gypsies (*koszos*) is not a Romanian word, but a Hungarian one. It is a rather general practice in Transylvania to sometimes use Hungarian words to convey some meanings that a seemingly equivalent Romanian word does not convey. Sandra uses the more extreme term *koszos* to express and ascribe a moral quality to the Romanies instead of the milder Romanian equivalent *murdar* (literally translatable as 'dirty').

3 This register of dirtiness, uncleanness, is all the more insidious as it is the backdrop of a collective, public, ideological representation of Romani people that positions them beyond reasonable bounds, beyond a civilized, orderly, moral order.

4 www.theguardian.com/uk-news/2013/nov/30/councils-home-office-begging-romanian-bulgarian.

5 See, for example, Vincze's (2013) compelling sociological analysis of socio-spatial marginality in the urban landfill of Cluj in Romania.

Chapter 7

Dehumanization and moral exclusion

In Chapter 6 I explored how various stories of transgression present Romani people as out of place. Romani people are described as people 'outside moral reach' (Bauman, 1990, p. 25), unworthy and undeserving of equal treatment. Talk of Roma as violators of pivotal social and moral conventions, as morally and spatially transgressive, delegitimizes their way of being in the world. For the majority of Europeans, regardless of their political leanings, Romani people are the embodiment of abjection, abhorrence and revulsion.

People, like the Roma, who are perceived as transgressors of moral (and spatial) boundaries, are typically classified as 'matter out of place'. In everyday talk the Roma are represented as uncanny (Kristeva, 1982), a dangerous, 'hovering presence' (Sibley, 1995). They are seen as carriers of symbolic danger and pollution, and as a consequence ought to be cast away from where orderly life is conducted and kept outside society's bounds. What is striking is how easy sympathy and reasonableness can be turned into delegitimizing and dehumanizing talk that alludes to Roma as residual, discardable, as something that needs purging, elimination and eradication. Obviously, eliminationist concerns are not something that can be proclaimed directly. Immoral tendencies must be kept at bay, under the veil of reasonableness.

In this chapter I consider the social psychology of dehumanization, defined as the implicit or explicit denial of humanity, dignity and humanness of people. I start by exploring dehumanization as a cognitive, as well as discursive and symbolic, process. I close the chapter by discussing some implications for researching societal and historical prejudices in general, and anti-Romani prejudices in particular, that stem from a close exploration of the collective, acceptable emotional canon of a community, where disgust is the foundation for reconfiguring, diminishing or denying people's worth and dignity.

Dehumanization as a cognitive process

Historical examples like the Nazi concentration camps, the horrors of Hiroshima, the Rwandan genocide, the massacres in Bosnia, etc., show that the humanity of human beings is not a given; they show that, under certain circumstances, the worth or dignity of *certain* people can be undermined, damaged, limited, with extreme consequences.

Traditionally, social psychologists have explored the humanity of human beings as something that can be operationalized, measured, quantified, by highlighting both positive and negative aspects. For instance, social psychologists have shown that thinking of 'all humanity' as our in-group can be a positive force for intergroup relations. This is social psychology's optimistic message grounded in its attempt to find a measurable and quantifiable indicator of the humanity of human beings. A more pessimistic message stems from the idea that humanness is a 'fundamental dimension of social perception' (Haslam and Loughnan, 2012, p. 91) and that restricting humanity to in-groups can have negative consequences for intergroup relations. In this section I focus on both the optimistic and pessimistic messages, with a greater emphasis on the latter.

One of the earliest attempts to find a measurable and quantifiable index of the humanity of human beings was Rosenberg's 1956 'Faith in People Scale'. The scale was believed to tap into beliefs regarding the trustworthiness, goodness and generosity of people in general. A more recent attempt is Luke and Maio's notion of 'humanity-esteem', which is defined as 'liking for people in general' (Luke and Maio, 2009).[1] Other researchers have considered the socio-psychological foundations of identification with 'all humanity', the factors that undermine it, as well as factors that might enhance it. McFarland's work (2010a, 2010b, 2011; McFarland and Brown, 2008) is an example of this. McFarland has designed the Identification With All Humanity Scale (IWAH) in order to tap into the notion of 'identification with all humanity'. The notion includes positive caring, a genuine concern and love for other human beings, and treating all other human beings as a part of one's in-group. As McFarland argues, 'we humans are not fated to categorize our social world only as ingroups and outgroups, or to think ethnocentrically. We are capable of thinking of *all humanity* as our ingroup, even if we rarely do so now' (2011, p. 16). Social problems, in McFarland's view, are '*humanity*'s problems, not national problems' (ibid.). McFarland's psychological message is interwoven with a cosmopolitan one. One must fight ethnocentrism and egocentrism (rather than considering them inevitable) because of their negative influence on 'our' identification with all humanity. McFarland's concern with identification with all humanity can be described in the terms of the 'omnicultural imperative' suggested by Moghaddam: 'during interactions with others, under all conditions, first give priority to the characteristics you share with other people as members of the human group' (2012, p. 318).

The reverse of this is a more pessimistic outlook. Categorizing our social world into in-groups and out-groups can have a negative effect on intergroup relations. Social psychologists have created a whole new vocabulary (e.g. 'infra-humanization', 'dehumanization', 'ontologization') for explaining what goes on when 'humanity' is restricted to in-groups (e.g. Leyens *et al.*, 2000, 2003; Paladino *et al.*, 2002 on infra-humanization; Bain *et al.*, 2013 on dehumanization; and Perez *et al.*, 2002 on ontologization).

For instance, 'infra-humanization' theory adopts a universalistic notion of 'being human' that emphasizes the role of essentially human attributes. One of the key insights of infra-humanization theory is the observation that each group member perceives his or her group as more 'human' than other groups. People tend to attribute secondary (uniquely human) emotions to their in-group and primary emotions to out-group members (Leyens *et al.*, 2000). According to Leyens and colleagues, 'both dominant and dominated groups can infra-humanize each other' (Leyens *et al.*, 2003, p. 706). Moreover, 'people infrahumanize the groups which they would not like or want to belong to' (Leyens, 2009, p. 813).

Research on 'dehumanization' proceeds from a distinction between 'human nature', described as characteristics 'essential or fundamental to all humans, such as openness, emotionality, vitality, and warmth' (Bastian *et al.*, 2011, p. 470), and 'human uniqueness', characteristics that 'distinguish humans from (other) animals, and involve refinement, civility, higher cognition, and other socially learned qualities' (ibid.). Researchers have observed experimentally how when 'human uniqueness' characteristics are denied to people, 'they are explicitly or implicitly likened to animals, and seen as immature, coarse, irrational, or backward' (ibid.).[2] The distinction between 'human nature' and 'human uniqueness' characteristics produces an operational definition of humanness, without which 'the concept of dehumanization is vague and slippery' (Haslam and Loughnan, 2012, p. 91). What some researchers call 'ontologisation' (Perez *et al.*, 2002) shares with 'infra-humanization' and 'dehumanization' an interest in an anthropological view of human nature and human 'essence'. The concept of 'ontologization' describes the psychological process that drives the representation of certain minorities (e.g. Gypsies) outside the realm of 'humanity'. According to the logic of 'ontologization', prejudice against out-groups is not only evaluative (that is, pertaining to negative evaluations and their discriminatory consequences), but also semantic-anthropological (the domain of 'ontologization') (cf. Marcu and Chryssochoou, 2005). The crux of 'ontologization' is that those perceived as Others (such as Romanies) are judged in terms of animal (natural), but not human (cultural) characteristics. It is argued that it is ultimately the anthropo-semantic cognitive process of 'ontologization' that leads to the 'inhuman' treatment of certain out-groups.

When social psychologists research 'ontologization', 'infra-humanization' or 'dehumanization', they place these concepts in a particular context – that of the psychological experiment. Experimental social psychology's conception of the humanity of human beings reflects the logico-scientific mode of thought. Research hypotheses produce 'working' definitions of humanness or humanity. These notions describe an intra-psychic dynamic. Notwithstanding their differences, the wealth of experiments on 'infra-humanization', 'dehumanization' and 'ontologization' show the 'growth of reliable experimental knowledge' (Chalmers, 1999, p. 209) on the humanity of human beings. There is an assumption that one cannot arrive at a deeper understanding of dehumanization simply by observing dehumanization as it naturally occurs in social situations, everyday social practices, in the media or in the public sphere more generally. There is a tendency amongst social psychologists to define the implicit or explicit denial of humanity, dignity and humanness of people as *what* experimental subjects accomplish/do in controlled experimental scenarios. Harré and Secord's classic evaluation of experimental research in psychology rings true:

> Psychologists, by and large, still believe that the way to clarify concepts is to invent experimental operations and to do experiments. They overlook the fact that such procedures, if they are to be used at all, have still to be linked up with social situations outside the laboratory, situations that are described by the subtle and enormously refined terms and concepts of ordinary language.
>
> (1972, p. 54)

Experiments on 'infra-humanization', 'dehumanization' and 'ontologization' remain at an operational level. There are virtually no attempts to research the broader phenomenon in an experiential or phenomenological sense. The notions of 'infra-humanization', 'dehumanization' or 'ontologization' are not derived from (nor do they index) an experiential domain; they are the outcome of an operational definition of human nature. Psychology's experimental descriptions of the humanity of human beings downplays the idea that these descriptions vary with time, place and observer, and they are the consequences of actual human experiences and encounters. Social psychologists' nomothetic explorations of humanity seem to derive 'more from the nature of the analysts' gaze than from what is gazed upon' (Reicher, 2004, p. 924).

Discursive and symbolic dehumanization

Although it is recognized that dehumanization undermines basic aspects of personhood – identity, self-determination, agency – and that is 'an interpersonally enacted and experienced phenomenon' (Bastian and Haslam, 2011, p. 302), there is less of a concern in social psychology with 'the actual complexes of activity and the actual processes of interaction in which human group life has its being' (Blumer, 1998 [1969], p. 138). Although it is acknowledged that everyday judgements of moral status are influenced by perceptions of humanness, there is no attempt to apply this reasoning to those social situations where perceptions of humanness have actual and real consequences for judgements of moral status, worth or dignity. In this section I explore the nature of everyday judgements of moral status, everyday judgements that alter or deny the humanity, dignity and humanness of people. I examine the symbolic and discursive actions, meanings and presuppositions that facilitate the denial of the humanity and dignity of Romanies, and highlight some of their societal consequences.

When researching dehumanization, psychology has turned its gaze away from the actual lives of people, their actual social practices, social interactions, representations and the contexts in which these appear (cf. Tileagă, 2013). As Billig (1994) has argued, psychology's pages are 'depopulated', devoid of what Allport has called 'concrete' human beings. Billig shows how psychologists often place a distance and tone of superiority between themselves and the people they are studying. Experiments and experimental controls render people 'passive and silent' (Reicher, 2011). As I have shown in the previous section, social psychologists construct and use an 'operational definition' of the general process of dehumanization and link it with specific 'procedures' for testing its existence. Operationalizing dehumanization means finding a measurable, quantifiable and valid index for it. Experimental research is engaged in a search for the *necessary* and *sufficient* conditions for the attribution and denial of humanity (Leyens, 2009).

But to search only for the necessary and sufficient conditions under which dehumanization operates at a psychological level would mean missing a fair share of its particular social and ideological aspects. In the laboratory, dehumanization is stripped of its social and ideological significance. It is presented as a universal and one-sided psychological process.[3] Its social and ideological significance comes into the foreground when researching dehumanization in real-world settings.[4]

When researching dehumanization in real-world settings the notion of dehumanization acquires a much wider meaning that encompasses issues to do with worth, dignity, moral status. In their attempt to make social psychology more relevant to the study of social issues and social problems, social psychologists should consider the myriad ways through which people construct, debate, assign or contest the humanity of others. When researching dehumanization, social psychologists should strive to use epistemologies and methodologies that are essential to researching 'social behaviour in its natural setting' (Harré and Secord, 1972, p. 44). Notions such as 'moral community', 'moral order', 'moral boundaries', 'moral inclusion' and 'moral exclusion' come to the fore when one attempts to research dehumanization and the social construction of extreme difference with reference to the lived discursive practices of everyday life. Whenever we are passing a judgement on the moral status of 'others' we are expressing societal moral meanings.

> [I]t is the society's appreciation or disdain of an individual's (norm-conforming or norm-breaking) behaviour that may change this individual's moral standing. This means, in a generalized mode, that whenever respect and approval (or disrespect and approval) for an individual are communicated, a moral discourse takes place (regardless of the feelings and thoughts of the participants).
>
> (Bergmann, 1998, p. 286)

In the remainder of this chapter I argue that, in order to understand the nature of delegitimizing and dehumanizing prejudices in general, and anti-Romani prejudices in particular, one needs to pay close attention to what people say, and the social context in which they place their moral discourses (Drew, 1998; Jayyusi, 1991; Linell and Rommetveit, 1998). In order to analyse what Tileagă (2007) calls 'ideologies of moral exclusion', one should look not merely for explicit, conventional and consensual, prejudiced tropes, but also for what is left unsaid and what is assumed to be beyond controversy (Billig, 1997).

In talking about Romanies, people are orienting to 'the boundaries between acceptable and non-acceptable opinion' (Billig, 1987, p. 133). In this chapter I use examples from Romanian majority-group members' interview talk that dehumanizes the Romanies (cf. also Tileagă, 2005, 2007). These illustrations come from individuals who support, are ambivalent towards or actively oppose exclusionary right-wing policies against minority groups. These are individuals who, routinely, see and present themselves as generally tolerant and open-minded.

As my argument so far has intimated, one need not turn to the 'hate speech' of professional extremists to find instances of talk that dehumanizes Romanies. The prejudices of the 'vast middle' describe Romanies as abhorrent, detestable, repulsive and unworthy of unequal treatment. These prejudices contain the seeds of ideological, eliminationist and genocidal discourses.

In Extract 7.1, Marta, a 48-year-old accountant, is invited to answer a question about the existence of discrimination against Romanies. Marta is not actively supporting the politics and policies of Romanian right-wing parties, yet she does not disavow them actively and directly either.

Extract 7.1

Chris Do you think that (.) there is much discrimination against
Romanies?
Marta There is no discrimination against Romanies, but there is
a revulsion=
Chris Hmm
(0.4)
Marta =it is a revulsion (.)and starting from this (0.4) it is
the state who is to blame (0.8) because for the Romanies,
the state gave importance, or priority to other ethnic groups,
and these were left (.) even though (.) even they
were also obligated to go to school and (.) until
1989 (0.8) it is a lack of education and probably it is
(1.2) their character of such nature (.) as a people (0.8)
as a people (.) but I don't understand why doesn't the
European Union accept them the way they are (.) So, why is
it only the Romanians that accept [the]m?
Chris [Hmm]
(0.4)
Marta °This I [don't] understand°
Chris [Do yo]u think that others want to get rid of them
Marta Yes, of course

A seemingly innocuous question about the existence of discrimination is answered through a direct and explicit denial of the existence of discrimination. The question presupposes a dimension of accountability of the majority group that Marta does not take up. Instead, the issue of majority-group accountability and negative reaction ('discrimination') is reframed, reformulated, as a different type of negative reaction ('revulsion'), with the onus shifting to Romanies. The repeated use of the extreme term 'revulsion' can be seen as a move towards establishing the out-there-ness of disgust. Marta's argument seems to be addressed to a 'universal audience' (Perelman and Olbrechts-Tyteca, 1971) to which the idea that the behaviour of Romanies is disgusting is non-controversial. It is a claim based on the implicit idea that everyone feels the same way (that is, disgusted) about the Romanies and their behaviour.

Marta's 'revulsion' remark implies a sense of Romanies as 'abject' (Kristeva, 1982), 'out of place', residual matter. Disgust is the emotion that triggers contempt. It is the quintessential emotional correlate of moral exclusion.

As others before her, Marta does not claim to be personally revolted by the Romanies; she portrays revulsion as a (reasonable) reaction independent of the feelings, wishes and motives of people. Hinting at revulsion as a reasonable response to Romanies' moral character is a common strategy used by speakers to deny moral legitimacy and equal moral standing in the world to Romanies, and place them in the realm of the aloof, detestable 'horror' (Jahoda, 1999).

Marta concedes that societal causes might account for the existence and persistence of prejudices against Romanies (ll. 498–500), yet she also volunteers a different kind of explanation that places the onus on consequences that derive from Romanies' moral character: 'it is a lack of education and probably it is (1) their character of such nature (.) as a people (0.8) as a people (.)' (ll. 502–504). Note the uncertainty move 'probably' and the implicit signs of difficulty (the scattered pauses), orientations to the sensitive and potentially extreme nature of her statement.

Marta closes her argument by invoking two seemingly rhetorical questions regarding the Romanies: 'why doesn't the European Union accept them the way they are (.) So, why is it only the Romanians that accept them? Interestingly, Marta's rhetorical questions echo the enduring protoconspirational mentality of participants who actively support right-wing policies against minorities. As several authors have argued (see, inter alia, Billig, 1987), the regularity of grammatical passive constructions and the asking of rhetorical questions inviting protoconspirational answers is a common strategy in the management of reasonableness in protoconspiratorial discourse.

But to explain what Marta is doing solely in terms of a protoconspirational mentality would be surely to miss the point and downplay the seriousness of her argument. I would argue that Marta uses the reference to the European Union as a warrant, a justification, for an implicit condemnation of Romanies on the basis of their moral character – 'the way they are' (l. 505). The premise of Marta's argument is that Romanies' moral character is problematic, yet socially forbidden wishes (wanting to 'get rid' of people) are distanced from the (national) self and attributed to others. Marta's response to the interviewer's attempt at clarification (ll. 510–511) reinforces this idea.

The possibility that 'we' (Romanians) might also wish to 'get rid' of Romanies cannot be uttered directly, and so is left unsaid. Marta's argument, which implicitly blames the Romanies for their predicament and dehumanizes them, is designed in such a way as to fend off any implications of inappropriate and immoral individual and collective socially forbidden, eliminationist desires.

What seems to be beyond controversy is the assumption that Romanies are, commonly, not wanted. This assumption is brought off collaboratively, with the interviewer playing his part in prompting Marta to emphasize the point. The collaborative claim about 'others' wanting to 'get rid of them' is in fact a double-claim (Billig, 1992), for 'we' (Romanians) are also implicitly hinted at. The Romanians' socially forbidden desires have been dropped out of the conversation. One can see how interviewer and interviewee are alluding to the possibility of immoral temptations and responses to Romanies' moral character, which are, however, routinely resisted and repressed.

The routine interaction in semi-structured interviews permits the operation of what Billig (1999) has called 'social repression'. Repression need not necessarily be understood in biological terms, if, as Billig contends, 'one assumes that socially inappropriate responses or thoughts, rather than biological urges, constitute the objects of repression' (ibid., p. 254). What is not said is as important as what is said. Subtle conversational avoidances and absences keep at bay socially immoral, socially unacceptable wishes and responses towards the Romanies.

Marta's seeming reasonableness hides a wider ideological struggle and moral tension between the requirements of a rational discourse of 'cultural' differences and an irrational, immoral eliminationist discourse. Here, as in many other cases of supposed reasonableness, there is a strong sense that there is something that cannot be directly stated. There is a repressed, unstated reference to 'us' (Romanians) harbouring socially forbidden desires as far as Romanies are concerned.[5]

As Kristeva (1982) argues, what (and *who*) is defined as abject is to be 'radically excluded', but is also, irrevocably, always a presence. Whatever (or whoever) is defined as abject can never be completely removed. As Marta and others like her argue, there seems to be a problem with the designation of a proper place for the Roma. Everyday language evocative of disgust and withdrawal from contact sets the stage for expressing ideas with eliminationist connotations.

In Extract 7.2, Alina, a 35-year-old accountant, is talking about the thorny issue of Roma integration in Romanian society. In contrast to Marta, Alina is a person who directly opposes and critiques the unreasonableness and unfairness of right-wing politics and policies against minorities. Yet, when it comes to talking about Romanies, her avowed tolerant, open-minded attitude shifts to diminishing Romanies' worth by using a language evocative of disgust and withdrawal from contact.

Extract 7.2

		(...)
413	Alina	I don't see the gypsies integrating themselves among us, they
414		don't like the civilized style[6] (.) by the way, they don't want to
415		go to school, they don't want at all to progress (.) I cannot have
416		an opinion about them (.) ha ha (.) but a bad one (.)
417	Chris	Whose blame it is, do you think?
418	Alina	Theirs, first of all, because I don't think (.) effectively, they
419		were dragged to school (.) they've been (.) they've been asked
420		to integrate and they cannot (.) There is at the end of Oradea,
421		I don't know where, a block especially built for them and (.) they
422		have eaten it from the ground like rats (.) isn't that so?
		(...)

Alina starts by admitting the unfeasibility of integration whilst being careful to offer appropriate justification for her position: 'they don't like the civilized style', 'they don't want to go to school', 'they don't want at all to progress' (ll. 413–415). Alina's justification draws upon some of the most commonly, widely shared tropes used to describe the moral inadequacy, and failure, of Romanies on key motivational schemes of society. Alina is at pains to provide a moral evaluation of Romanies' societal worth by using what discursive psychologists call 'dispositional talk' (Edwards, 2003). As argued in Chapter 6, disposition formulations (not *wanting*, not *liking* to do certain things) are ways in which whatever one is saying about the Romanies has to do with their moral character. Disposition formulations are ways of 'fixing' Romanies' non-normative behaviour in their moral character. Dispositional formulations permit the expression of socially shared, recognizable, negative portrayals of Romani people, whilst fending off the opprobrium of a prejudiced identity. Alina uses disposition formulations to construct a contrast between Romani backwardness and inadequacy, and normative societal values and assumptions.

Alina's talk echoes firm and established societal tropes that describe Romanies as constantly failing the various (normative) tests of worth that society imposes on them. The reference to 'civilization', and 'civilized' behaviour, which Romanies fail to observe, diminishes Romanies' worth and positions them as marginal, outside a normative moral order. As Dixon *et al.* (1997) point out, 'the category "civilized" relies on that which is banished beyond its threshold' (p. 342).[7]

The full implication of Alina's dispositional talk is revealed several lines later. The story of impropriety and transgression that Alina offers at lines 420–422 brings, again, the issue of Romanies' worth to the forefront. This is not a typical story of transgression, but one that implies aspects that cannot be uttered directly. Notice the extreme reference to 'rats', which dehumanizes

Romanies and presents them as vermin. This representation of 'people', 'human beings' as animals, 'as particular species which are associated with residues or the borders of human existence' (Sibley, 1995, p. 27), achieves a relegation of Romanies to the status of the abject and denies their 'human' qualities. Romanies are associated with 'dirt' and an insidious register of impurity. Rats are filthy animals, which need to be eliminated for cleanliness. As dirt has to be removed from 'our' houses, likewise, people categorized as 'dirt' are to be removed from 'civilized' society. This extreme description has clear eliminationist connotations. Rats are carriers of terrible diseases, in the same way as Romanies are carriers of an ultimate threat to moral order, which must be eliminated.[8]

Talking on the same subject several lines later, Alina justifies further her indignation by using eliminationist imagery.

Extract 7.3

```
        (...)
Alina   What can society do for them? (.) To make them a communal bath,
        they destroy it (.) it builds them a block (.) it is destroyed
        (.) No, you cannot take it with them, it is something like (.) like
        (.) the scum (.) the scum of society, how should I put it (mm)
```

The opening rhetorical question ('What can society do for them?') sets the Romani ***problem*** as an issue without a ***solution***. It is implied that there is nothing that ('our') society can do for them. The implication is that the Romanies are *the* problem, a problem, that is, to the rest of society (notice the factuality of her descriptions at ll. 428–429). Although the problem is formulated (in strong terms), the solution is unformulated. Being cast as the 'problem' that calls for a solution, Romanies are not regarded as moral subjects on an equal footing. Romanies are being denied the status of moral objects and subjects, the power of 'moral command' (Bauman, 1990), an autonomous moral standing and worth in 'our' (civilized, settled, normative) world. The problematic nature of Romanies' moral character hints at a solution outside the bounds of democratic and moral procedure.

At lines 430–431, Alina is in search of a formulation that could capture her previous description, and the general feeling about Romanies: 'the scum of society'. A metaphor of residue stands as a metaphor for residual people. To categorize Romanies as residual, as abject par excellence, is, again, to ignore their visible human qualities and autonomous worth, and to allude to a conclusion with eliminationist connotations. All the premises for an eliminationist conclusion are in place, yet it is something that cannot be directly stated.[9]

There is a call for an implicit solution. Evidence is presented that rational solutions to the 'problem' have not worked, and that by implication there is no rational solution to deal with 'them'. In such circumstances of delegitimizing and dehumanizing talk, immoral and socially forbidden desires lurk under the surface. The immoral, eliminationist conclusion is implicitly contained in the premises. What is not said, what is absent from the interaction cannot nevertheless be absent from the analysis. The repression of immorality, what is not said (but could easily have been), becomes of central importance.

Arguably, Alina like Marta before her does not express an individual attitude, but rather a collective attitude, firmly entretched in common sense, that constructs and perpetuates the acceptability of societal tropes and frameworks, that diminish, transform or deny Romanies' moral worth. This is a collective attitude that says that the worth, dignity, of people is derived from staunch loyalty to the moral values and motivational schemes of the majority group and society. Anyone found not to be adhering to, or following, the values and motivational schemes of society will have their worth diminished or denied. Following the steps of Freud, Billig cogently argues that 'immorality always lurks on the edge of overdemanding morality' (1997, p. 148). When talking about Romanies, right-thinking and self-righteous citizens are stopping short of uttering the unsayable.

Across the political spectrum, a discourse of delegitimization and dehumanization is used to portray the Romanies as matter 'out of place', as polluting our moral and physical space, an ultimate 'threat' for which a (radical) solution is needed. Socially forbidden desires (wishes for a radical solution) lurk under the surface of supposed reasonablencss and tolerant identities. The dialogue between interviewer and interviewee creates its own unsaid matters: 'if conscious thought is shaped by rhetoric, then so might the dynamics of dialogue provide the resources for repression' (Billig, 1998, p. 206).

Social repression is enacted in relation to a specific *category of people* that 'we', the settled, the civilized, etc., categorize as matter 'out the place', as abject, as deplorable. Social repression comes into play when 'solutions' to this 'problem' are implicitly felt to fall outside the bounds of democratic and moral procedure. As Billig has claimed, social repression is something that is 'part of ideological and socio-historical currents' (1997, p. 152). Understanding the dynamics of social repression might help in understanding what might be repressed in the European contemporary cultural climate, but also in relation to *whom*.

Violence, disgust and the emotional capital of intolerance

The explicit, dehumanizing collective tropes that are used to talk about Romanies point in the direction of an ideological and historical tradition of persecution of Romanies. This tradition of persecution includes both discursive and non-discursive aspects. One of the most tangible manifestations of a tradition of persecution is violence. Under certain conditions, dehumanizing talk can turn into, or facilitate, dehumanizing violence.

The tangible contemporary manifestations of violence against Romanies in Europe (see Amnesty International, 2014 for a very recent and comprehensive report) show that violence is a manifestation less of individual, irrational mindsets, than of collective, ruling-state institutions and policies (like the police) whose aim is to uproot what they see as the wretched face of poverty, lawlessness and transgressive and immoral behaviour. Violence against the Roma is a concrete, special type of violence – it is what might be called uprooting, deracinating violence (burning Roma houses down or dismantling makeshift camps); it is violence that gives Romanies a clear signal that they are not wanted. Social psychologists need to start considering carefully how uprooting violence is experienced by individuals and communities, the consequences of this type of violence (and its sometimes subtle forms), as well as the various societal factors that might trigger it. Uprooting violence presupposes three types of moral exclusion working in concert: 'exclusion within society' (forced relocation, discrimination in employment, etc.); 'exclusion from society' (homes destroyed, forced repatriation, etc.); and 'exclusion as annihilation' (death, murder) (cf. Opotow, 2011).[10]

The community of right-thinking and self-righteous citizens that condemn the Roma, that find the Roma out of place, disgusting and horrible by the standards of civilized society, is not only a community of values, but is also what Rosenwein (2006) has called an 'emotional community'. Any emotional community trades in emotional capital – the positive, progressive emotions of tolerance (compassion, empathy) and the negative emotions of intolerance (abhorrence, disgust).

Both discursive and material, tangible reflections of a tradition of persecution are steeped in a form of emotional capital where expressing disgust is acceptable. Disgust is perhaps the most visible form of affect used in accounting for Roma's worth and moral status. In accounts of moral transgression, accounts that describe the Roma as violators of pivotal norms of civilized behaviour, disgust is affect performed publicly. Disgust is a form of affect that carries a message about the worth of people. Disgust mingles with anxiety and contempt. Disgust is widely seen as an acceptable form of emoting. As this chapter has shown, people do not express personal disgust but rather point to the reasonableness of being disgusted by the presence, behaviour, way of being, of Romanies. Disgust is a central part of the emotional capital of a community of right-thinking, self-righteous citizens that find Romanies inadequate, not worthy of equal treatment. Groups, communities and societies are carriers of emotional capital – tolerance and empathy, as well as intolerance. Sanctioned ways of talking about Others reflect the diversity, depth or shallowness of emotional capital. Emotional registers of tolerance, empathy, openness, open-mindnesses (positive social emotions) coexist with registers of intolerance, lack of empathy, disgust and withdrawal from contact.

Politicians, representatives of local government, usually stir, frame and reframe the emotional capital of their communities, societies and nations, especially when discussing social problems. The presence of social problems (usually those that result from the actions of those perceived as Others, like immigration or spatial transgression, for instance) constitutes the perfect background for the rehearsal and creative reinvention of existing and new emotional capital. Emotional capital interweaves with social and political cultural capital; that is, all those ways of talking, and taken-for-granted values and practices that allow societies, groups and communities to reproduce themselves as certain kinds of societies. Emotional capital of a community, or nation, contains all those affective practices that give a nation its affective 'habitus'. These are affective practices that enact tolerance and/or intolerance.

In the case of intolerance and dehumanizing practices, disgust becomes part of the acceptable 'affective canon' that characterizes the community of the unworthy. The European recession, intra-European migration, the new faces of poverty, have revived a forgotten, repressed affective canon of intolerance. They not only allowed it to resurface, but also made it increasingly acceptable. An acceptable affective canon of intolerance becomes 'woven together in subtle ways with people's usual communal methods for describing, accounting for, and judging self and others' (Wetherell, 2012, p. 116). Disgust is only one aspect of an affective canon of intolerance, but is perhaps the most pernicious, especially when it mingles with contempt, derision and humiliation of a certain, very specific category of people.

When part of an acceptable emotional canon of a community, disgust is a platform for reconfiguring people's worth and interpersonal and intergroup relations. Disgust is a special type of affective practice; one needs to construct grounds for being disgusted; one cannot do it as an individual, one needs to imagine oneself as belonging to a community that feels the same way (that is, disgusted) in relation to a specific group of people. As affective practice, disgust cannot be satisfactorily described as simply rooted in psycho-evolutionary (Schaller and Neuberg, 2012) or neural (Harris and Fiske, 2006) dynamics. Disgust is a collective affective practice. It is the emotional *appui* for a communal representation of people who are perceived as failures on the moral schemes of neoliberal democracies. It matters less whether those who are disgusted by the Roma are Romanian, French, Italian or British; what they all agree upon is that the Roma ought to be treated differently; and, indeed, where they differ is in their differential treatment of the Roma.

As collective affective practice, disgust denies value, dignity, to people or communities perceived as unworthy, lesser human types. Like other affective practices, disgust is a means to 'construct and mark boundaries' (Wetherell, 2012, p. 114) and is a precursor to action. Disgust, expressed even by the most tolerant members of European societies, is an implicit call to action. It calls for the containment of the threat of contamination or pollution, it calls for the removal, physical exclusion and obliteration of anything that upsets order, whilst ignoring the affective practices of those classed as Others, and their own reactions to humiliation, displacement and alienation.

The emotional capital of disgust counters and stifles the emotional capital of minority group (Roma) emancipation. Psychological (and moral) distance is an outcome of the dynamics of collective emotional capital. Although, in theory, liberal democratic societies are structured along the lines of human commonalities (Moghaddam, 2012) and the creation, preservation and protection of superordinate identities, in practice, liberal democratic societies fail to give full airing to the emotional capital of the emancipation of Roma themselves. The language of EU roadmaps for Roma emancipation is telling in this respect. Although the voice of the Roma is represented, the affective register is limited to the emotional capital of majority-group or European priorities, with the Roma accountable for their own predicament and full and unconditional 'integration'. The values of the Roma, and their own emotional capital, are recognized, but subtly downgraded. It is left to Roma activists to search for the most appropriate form of emotional capital that would allow them to open and sustain a more systematic dialogue with Europe and its collective values. European policy ushers everyone into a new era of cohesion and diversity, as the national and global challenges of our time (Cantle, 2008), yet individuals, groups and communities across Europe continue to perceive Romanies as unworthy of equal treatment. Individuals, groups and communities across Europe reproduce what Honneth has called 'evaluative forms of disrespect' that imply the 'denigration of individual or collective ways of life' (1996, p. 134).

Dehumanizing talk, and other manifestations of moral exclusion, are thus not a problem of antipathy or irrational individual psychology. As I have tried to show in this chapter, they are more a matter of drawing upon a collective, acceptable 'affective canon' that portrays and reproduces, subtly or explicitly, an ideology of Roma as 'out of place' and repulsive. Dehumanizing talk denies public recognition of someone's dignity and social and moral worth. It removes Romanies from the domain of moral acceptability and prepares the ground for uprooting violence.

Prejudices of the 'vast middle' are not automatic, or unconscious, they are not lodged in people's psyches but rather are evaluative prejudices – they transform and shape the degree of social and moral esteem, and social approval, of a specific category of people within the boundaries of a self-righteous, self-sufficient moral collective. Depriving people of social esteem and social approval means depriving them of their humanity, presenting them as less than human. Prejudices of the 'vast middle' contain the seeds of eliminationist discourses, continually repressed and inhibited by the requirements of righteous morality.

The contemporary European challenge is how to treat others who are alike, but also, essentially, unlike 'us'. Social psychologists should be able to explore how individuals, groups and communities address this challenge without exclusive recourse to individual psychology, but through a focus on social practices, collective assumptions, that facilitate the refusal of autonomous moral standing and worth in the world to those perceived and described as, essentially, unlike 'us'.

Notes

1 Luke and Maio argue that 'humanity-esteem' is a global measure that reflects 'emotions toward people, stereotypes of people, and symbolic beliefs about people' (2009, p. 588). High levels of 'humanity-esteem' are seen as a robust predictor of reduced social conflict.
2 When 'human nature' attributes are denied to people 'they are explicitly or implicitly likened to objects or machines and seen as cold, rigid, inert, and lacking emotion' (Bastian *et al.*, 2011, p. 470).
3 Interestingly, psychological concepts like 'infra-humanization' or 'ontologization' do not seem to have an opposite. There is a certain one-sidedness to such concepts. A single cognitive process is considered without equal weight being given to an opposing counter-process (Billig, 1991).
4 Dehumanization might be that area of social behaviour for the deeper understanding of which we 'may … need to abandon the laboratory for the actual world' (Harré and Secord, 1972, p. 50).
5 Moreover, as Billig (2002a) observes, 'what is socially forbidden can become an object of desire and pleasure. If there are taboos on the expression of bigotry in contemporary society, outward prejudice may take the form of a forbidden pleasure. Bigotry, then, becomes a temptation' (p. 185).
6 Civilized lifestyle.
7 Bauman's (1995) comments on how 'we' – the 'normal', 'civilized' people – deal with the 'danger-carrying strangers' (p. 179) acquire significance in this context. As he argues, 'we throw the carriers of danger up and away from where the orderly life is conducted; we keep them out of society's bounds' (ibid., p. 180).
8 In their analysis of anti-Semitism, Adorno *et al.* (1982 [1950]) make reference to the power and ideological consequences of eliminationist imagery. For example, there is mention of 'the metaphor of the rotten apple in the barrel [that] conjures up the imagery of "evil germs" which is associated with appalling regularity with the dream of an effective germicide' (p. 653).
9 Whilst the consequences of Romani behaviour and way of being in the world are presented as morally problematic, the consequences of Alina's eliminationist categorization are not. This is not surprising, as Edelman argues, since members of the civilized, fair-minded, tolerant society are not inclined to raise ethical issues that imply that 'this fine group of ours, with its humanitarianism and its high-minded principles might be capable of adopting a course of action that is inhumane and immoral' (1977, p. 94).
10 What these three types of exclusion bring into play is a collective attitude that presupposes that 'those excluded from the scope of justice are seen as: psychologically distant, undeserving of constructive obligations, and eligible for harms that would be unacceptable for those inside the scope of justice' (Opotow, 2011, p. 207).

Chapter 8

Towards a critical social psychology of racism

One of the most serious questions that social psychologists of racism are asking is also, perhaps, the simplest too: 'why can't we just get along?' (Dovidio *et al.*, 2002b). It is the type of concern that seems to be at the core of modern scientific analyses of racism. But it is not only a contemporary concern. A similar concern can be found in the classic studies of the discipline. For instance, Myrdal has expressed it aptly too: 'why all ... potentially and intentionally good people so often make life a hell for themselves and each other when they live together, whether in a family, a community, a nation or a world' (Myrdal, 1996 [1944], p. 1023).

The *just* in 'why can't we just get along?' points to the idea that normal expectations of 'getting naturally along' are not met. Dovidio and colleagues suggest that there is a good reason why 'we can't just get along' – it is because there is something about the nature of racism that hinders the promotion and internalization of values such as communication, trust or solidarity. Communication and trust are 'critical to developing long-term positive intergroup relations' (Dovidio *et al.*, 2002b, p. 89), but (aversive) racism, in tandem with subtle, unconscious biases foster miscommunication and distrust. The question of 'why can't we just get along' is not only a question about specific groups (e.g. white and black Americans as in the case of Dovidio *et al.*); it is a universal question that can easily be applied to other contexts.

It is a question that cannot be answered without pondering the nature of racism in society. Social psychologists tend to attribute the complexity of contemporary racism to subtle, unconscious bias. Although this is a very influential and rich avenue of inquiry, it offers only a partial answer. Subtle bias can get in the way of interpersonal and intergroup sympathy, solidarity and mutual trust, but arguably, it is only one aspect that can explain the complexity of racism in society. One cannot understand the nature and complexity of racism in society without exploring the nature of (specific) societies, social and institutional arrangements, societal values, collective assumptions and presuppositions, which perpetuate intolerance as well as tolerance.

The American conversation about 'getting along' to which Dovidio and colleagues allude is presumably different from European conservations on the moral status that should be assigned to Romanies in European societies. Turning to societies' conversations about and with themselves might reveal a much broader spectrum of societal, non-psychological aspects that participate in the situated genesis, perpetuation and collective definition of prejudice.

If prejudice is truly an interpretive concept then we should perhaps pay more attention to the genesis, perpetuation and collective definition of prejudice in specific (national and transnational) socio-cultural contexts. In a Europe that tries to protect its citizens from what European politicians call the 'undesirable effects of globalization', a desire to uphold the values of sympathy coexists with a desire to control the flux of people, erect barriers and enforce boundaries. In this climate, toughness and conservatism coexist with reasonableness and humanitarianism. European liberal democracies are mechanisms of domination as well as empowerment (Fassin, 2005). In Europe the question of 'why can't we just get along' is intimately linked to the matter of the moral status that should be assigned to others who are alike, but also, fundamentally, unlike 'us'. This matter, in turn, cannot be addressed without reflecting on the tension between two Europes: a cosmopolitan Europe that struggles against ethnocentric temptations (Beck, 2006) and a conservative Europe, attempting to protect what it sees as its 'patrimony', but careful to champion a rhetoric of human values and sympathy (Finkielkraut, 2013).

The critical analysis of intolerance and decent society

None of the perspectives I examined in this book is satisfactory alone. The answer to the quandaries posed by the study of anti-Roma prejudices does not lie in the similarities or differences that divide the various schools of thought or methodological choices. The answer 'must be sought in characteristics of society that affect us all, whatever our methodological or theoretical persuasion' (Becker, 1967, p. 239). These characteristics include a society's creed and form of social organization, social norms and also assumptions about justice, dignity, decency, fairness and equal treatment of people, welfare, or solidarity. In this book I argued that we need a broader analytical framework to be able to account satisfactorily for the scope and complexity of subtle and blatant prejudices, which includes (but is not limited to) the exploration of the, sometimes paradoxical, clash between progressive social creeds and values and actual discriminatory, and moral exclusionary, practices.

In Chapter 1 I outlined three lines of argument that make up the core of a critical analysis of racism. I will only briefly recapitulate them here.

First, prejudice, racism and discrimination are social and cultural creations. Discursive, symbolic and material practices create and perpetuate prejudice, racism and discrimination. These practices are sourced in the complex and contradictory social imaginary of societies, and in the ways in which individuals, groups and communities recognize or alter, transform, diminish, each other's moral worth. Second, as social and cultural creations, prejudice, racism and discrimination are tied to the inherent tension between democratic modes of domination and sympathy, control and compassion (Fassin, 2005). Finally, social psychologists need to be able to mobilize methodological stances that are appropriate to researching prejudice as a social and cultural creation, and to capturing the foundational tension between democratic modes of domination and sympathy, control and compassion. Methods (and concepts) should be derived from a focus on social problems and public conversations around social problems.

We have a lot to learn from researching prejudice in what ethnographers and anthropologists call 'field situations'; we have a lot to learn about prejudice by analysing data generated in and by cultural spheres. For instance, in Chapter 4 I have argued that ethnographies of identity are much more powerful tools in the hands of social scientists than assumed or imagined models of identity. Ethnography can capture both objective and subjective aspects of Roma identity. They can reveal aspects of identity categories that would remain invisible to conventional approaches to identity. They also show that identity categories are sourced in the complex and symbolic social imaginary of societies. Ethnographers can describe a varied anthropological world of people and social relations that are not necessarily tied to psychological mental processes. Social psychologists should follow suit, and become more skilled at describing, and interpreting, everyday occurrences of categories, especially those that are used for intergroup as well as intragroup differentiation.

In this book I highlighted the uniqueness and particularity, the diversity and intensity, of anti-Romani prejudices as an example of one of the most troubling contemporary social problems for European societies. I, hopefully, showed how little can be explained with reference to (subtle, automatic, unconscious) inner mental processes or personality, and what can be gained by considering broader societal aspects around the worth and the dignity of people, and the prejudices of the self-righteous and right-thinking 'vast middle'.

Critical analysis explores heuristic avenues that open a dialogue between social psychology and cognate fields – anthropology, social theory and sociology. Social visions and intellectual strands in these fields can be used to strengthen and reorient a renewed social psychology of racism (Boltanski, 2012; Fassin, 2005; Wacquant, 2008). Critical analysis can inform both universalist and relativist social psychological approaches to prejudice. Analysis is 'critical' insofar as it addresses societal dilemmas, tensions, contradictions (of tolerance and intolerance), that are hidden in plain view.

A critical analysis of racism takes the form of a cultural analysis of society, its presuppositions, repertoires, discursive and social practices that offend and degrade or transform and diminish the worth of individuals and communities. Any critical analysis of racism needs to take into account the societal (discursive, historical, anthropological/symbolic and socio-structural) 'life-space' of prejudice (cf. Moscovici, 2011).[1] A critical analysis is a cultural, in-depth analysis of how a society accomplishes itself as a *decent* society, how it reconciles a desire for order and compassion couched in a language of respectability. In today's Europe, decent societies can be said to rely on

> a strong and active (but not brutally 'domineering') state and a vigorous and innovative (but not recklessly 'liberated') capitalist economy as powerful means in the challenge of engaging all citizens and all communities in the task of living together without poverty and humiliation.
> (Smith, 2006, p. 201)

The primary aim of a critical analysis of racism is to understand how decent societies operate, what values and principles they use to regulate processes of inclusion and exclusion, the positive and negative argumentative spaces and consequences these values and principles generate, and the actual and potential contradictions between declarations of decency and actual treatment of people.

From antipathy to indignity

Critical analysis opens the way for a meaningful, and transformed, social psychology of racism that can establish itself more as sociology and anthropology, rather than a psychology, of modern democratic culture. Critical analysis shifts the onus of social psychological analyses of prejudice: from prejudice as an attitudinal product of antipathy to prejudice as harm inflicted by indignity. It also urges social psychologists to base their analyses on a more explicit, metatheory of society (as a reflexive product of discursive, symbolic and material orders and practices), with roots in sociological and anthropological theory. This is a framework particularly suited to researching what Allport called 'stubborn' prejudices. Europeans seem to agree on the *existence* of a social problem, but they disagree on the *moral nature* of the 'problem' that Romanies pose. Deciding on the moral nature of the problem that Roma pose to European society involves a collective conversation about the *worth*, *place* and *fate* of Romanies in Europe. The explicitly declared European creed of law, justice, security and freedom for all, clashes with concrete practices that exclude, debase, degrade people, yet it remains implicit, and passes unnoticed. Western and Eastern European societies are, more than ever before, conducting such conversations about the worth, place and fate of Romanies in Europe. These are conversations about the limits of solidarity, sympathy and compassion in liberal democracies; conversations about how to alter, transform or diminish the worth of people who are seen as failures according to the moral schemes of liberal democratic society.

The idea of prejudice as explicit or implicit bias only partly describes and explains the direction and intensity of prejudices and the uniqueness of targets of prejudice. As I argued in the Introduction to this book, history, as well as research, shows that not all prejudices are the same: they are culturally and ideologically situated, their expression depends on a complex interplay of socio-cultural, political and ideological factors. Portraying anti-Roma prejudices as fundamentally a psychological problem restricts the critical reach of questions that can be asked. Social psychologists should be able to describe, and offer explanations for, both subtle and blatant/extreme prejudices without unique recourse to individual psychology. If prejudice *is* and *does* something, as Allport argues, then it is insufficient to research it as a 'basic psychological problem' (Allport, 1954). If prejudice is and does something, if it hurts and harms people, if it degrades and dehumanizes people, then it should also be studied as a basic problem of collective definition (Tileagă, 2014), that is to say, a basic problem of defining the boundaries of common social experience.

Collective definitions of common social experience impact on how we define dignity, respect and worth of citizens and of people defined as Others. Contemporary European discrimination against Romanies (and the resulting inequalities) is based on assigned extreme differences of social esteem and dignity. 'Tests' of worth (Boltanski and Thévenot, 2006 [1991]), especially created for aliens, refugees and strangers, stifle, distort and diminish the public recognition of someone's dignity and social worth. When we talk or write about dignity, we are alluding to an individual's or group's right 'to be acknowledged publicly as what they already really are' (Appiah, 1994, p. 149). If, as I suggested in the Introduction, prejudice is harm inflicted by indignity, then a social psychology of racism should include amongst its concerns an account of how people's *worth* is modified, altered, and the consequences of such modifications. Both deliberate (and more subtle) attempts at altering, transforming, diminishing the worth of Romanies refuses them the social esteem and moral status that other people (other groups) take for granted.

Discourses and practices that remove Romanies from the domain of moral acceptability (both physically and symbolically) can have pernicious as well as subtler, long-term consequences. The idea of prejudice as indignity is not just about the forms and consequences of extreme forms of social hostility. It is also about understanding the less noticeable, ambivalent, paternalistic, social and ideological ramifications of refusal/denial of dignity as a product of modern democratic society.

It would be a mistake to attribute the inexcusable treatment of Romanies in France, Italy or Great Britain solely to hostility. As I argued in this book, the Roma embody the new face of marginality (and poverty) that occasions moral-political dilemmas, stirs deep-seated passions and unsettles the conventional, democratic negotiation of social problems. This new face of marginality (and poverty) upsets the tolerant and inclusive image that liberal democracies construct of themselves. As I argued in Chapter 6, evictions, isolation of Roma in ghettos or slums or removal from city centres carry a sizeable weight of dishonour (Wacquant, 2008) that enhances individual, group and community feelings of indignity.

Solidarity, sympathy and European civilized opinion

In liberal democratic societies the line separating dignity from indignity is precarious. The instances of anti-Roma racism recounted in this book point to the idea that racism is not simply a matter of negative attitudes and/or flawed psychology. Allport also recognized that prejudices are a 'prime source of suffering and disvalue' (Allport, 1960, p. 225). Researching prejudices as a source of disvalue implies researching public, not private, prejudices, especially those prejudices whose consequences take the form of an explicit or implicit attempt to transform or diminish people's social esteem and worth.

Understanding the crux of anti-Roma prejudices, as source of suffering and disvalue, presupposes understanding the nature of solidarity and sympathy in liberal democracies and the nature of civilized opinion as a contradictory social mixture.

The illustrations contained in this book, albeit limited in scope, show that solidarity and sympathy are not guaranteed by being enshrined in the European or national constitutions. Rather they are *conditional* and *ambiguous*, insufficient values for the protection of human dignity. The idea of 'equal human dignity' is enshrined in many national and international charters, but, in practice, dignity/indignity take complex forms and manifestations. As I argued in Chapter 7, one major source of indignity is disgust, the political emotion that, as Nussbaum (2013) argues, 'blocks equal political respect' (p. 186). Disgust, as social evaluation, replaces sympathy and solidarity as responses to injustice in decent societies. Disgust, as 'a key device of subordination' (ibid., p. 182), goes hand in hand with the taboo of contact, and blocks the expression of genuine solidarity and sympathy.[2]

Disgust is a relational social and political emotion. The expression of disgust is dependent on acceptable social forms of evaluative responses in society. By withdrawing solidarity and sympathy, Romanies are not only actively degraded by societies, they are also constantly reminded of their modified worth and degraded status. European civilized opinion does not seem to find an appropriate moral-evaluative response for the dignity of Romanies. In its most basic form, indignity is the 'rejection of a person from the human commonwealth' (Margalit, 1998, p. 3) and the loss of control over one's own destiny and means of self-definition. As Taylor (1994, p. 25) argues,

> a person or group of people can suffer real damage, real distortion, if the people or society around them mirror back to them a confining or demeaning or contemptible picture of themselves. Nonrecognition or misrecognition can inflict harm, can be a form of oppression, imprisoning someone in a false, distorted, and reduced mode of being.

European civilized opinion that demeans and degrades Romanies is, however, a contradictory social mixture, where ethnocentric instincts, and desire for control and protection of national essences, coexist with the reflective criticism of sympathetic cosmopolitanism or compassionate conservatism. European civilized opinion supports the value of a 'more inclusive conception of the European polity based on recognition and solidarity' (Delanty, 2009, p. 202), yet, at the same time, refuses it to Romanies.

European civilized opinion is made up of the vast majority of right-thinking and well-intentioned European citizens that perceive the rise of the extreme right as one of the core challenges to a cosmopolitan, more open and more inclusive Europe. The sources of extreme right-wing sentiment are usually located in social malaise, corruption of traditional values, fear and threat. Extreme views are said to reflect the irrational responses of a, psychologically insecure, minority. Yet, when the same right-thinking and well-intentioned citizens talk about Romanies they reproduce, uncritically and unthinkingly, extremist tropes, degrading and dehumanizing repertoires that transform or diminish Romanies' moral standing in society. European civilized opinion comprises well-intentioned prejudices that rehearse degrading, debasing, dehumanizing descriptions of people.

Social justice and post-racism

European civilized opinion extends to what might be called well-intentioned European institutions as well. Major European think tanks are tasked with delivering social justice: solving the 'problems' of integration, the negative consequences of poverty, destitution, unemployment and inequalities of health and gender. The situation of Romanies is deplored, but also recognized as very difficult to change. It is the urgent goal of these institutions to remove inequality whilst 'civilizing' Romanies, therefore giving priority to eliminating societal ills over ensuring everyday respect for some of its more vulnerable members. It is believed that respect, dignity, will follow, will be a by-product, of the elimination of societal ills. The agenda of 'inclusion' and 'exclusion' has been replaced by the agendas of 'cohesion' and 'diversity' as challenges that face Europe in response to processes of globalization. 'Poverty', 'destitution', 'unemployment', 'healthcare', 'housing', etc., have replaced racism on the agenda of European policy-makers. Racism is perceived as a pernicious effect or consequence of a failure of managing community cohesion and diversity.

European policy for the Roma frames its progressive actions in a post-racism era. Although racism still persists, it is presented as a thing of the past; a progressive, globalized Europe does not protect racism and racists. Yet, infringements of core European values and principles, like freedom of movement or settlement, are not always perceived as racist. European elites can freely castigate new member countries for failing to integrate their Roma populations, whilst at the same time reproducing explicitly an ideology of Roma as 'out of place'. In an interview for Mittelweg, Jacques Delors argued recently that

> we ought to be telling Bulgaria and Romania to get on with the social integration of the Roma, using the money that the Commission has earmarked for that objective, or else they will be handed a red card. Having said that, the way that the Roma are treated in France and Italy is no less scandalous. Of course, the Roma cannot go just anywhere but to conclude from that that it is acceptable to destroy the places where they live and force them to return to Romania or Bulgaria is scandalous.
>
> (Tietze and Bielefeld, 2010)

Politicians, like Delors, can display indignation at the treatment of Roma by established liberal democracies, whilst at the same time highlighting explicitly Roma's moral transgression. As I argued in Chapter 6 the idea that 'the Roma cannot just go anywhere' is a very powerful notion that is used to keep the Roma in a subordinate position, and is used to justify harsh treatment. People who are denied freedom of movement and settlement are denied dignity. Romanies' free movement in Europe is presented as unruly; they are causing problems that nation-states have to solve. Delors advocates the voice of the new, 'planned' democracy of the European Union that presents itself as a progressive project of inclusivity, social justice and firm accountability, yet rehearses uncritically moral exclusionary discourses.

The sympathetic cosmopolitanism of inclusion coexists with pragmatic, economic visions. The first EU legal instrument for Roma inclusion outlines the stakes of Roma integration in Europe:

> Roma integration is not only a moral duty, but in the interest of Member States, especially for those with a large Roma minority. Roma represent a significant and growing proportion of the school age population and the future workforce. Efficient labour activation policies and individualised and accessible support services for Roma job seekers are crucial to allow Roma people to realise their hu.man capital and to actively and equally participate in the economy and society.
>
> (European Council, December 2013)

Although the document positions the realization of Roma's 'human capital' as a key emancipatory value, it does not also highlight the barriers that

Roma are facing when trying to participate in the European dream of an organic economic community, which has to respond to vast, varied and complex individual, social and economic needs. Presenting Roma as the future European workforce ignores the difficulties they are facing in the present. It places the onus on the Roma and the need to change, whilst ignoring their diversity and multifarious needs. What the policy documents do not stipulate are the potentially harsh moral consequences for not cooperating. The rhetoric of economic pressures and challenges outlines and proposes tests of worth, which not all Roma may pass. The contemporary struggle of European societies with 'cohesion' and 'diversity' is constituted by attempts to make Romanies a bit more 'like us'.

In the name of 'inclusive sympathy' (Nussbaum, 2013, p. 2), integration proceeds top-down. A national and European philosophy of pragmatism that relies on a 'gubernatorial-bureaucratic style' of juridification (Habermas, 2012) indicates the requirements of clear and strict accountability. Take, for instance, the words of Vice-President Viviane Reding, the EU Justice Commissioner, on the European Council's legal instrument for Roma inclusion:

> Today's agreement is a strong signal that Member States are willing to tackle the challenging task of Roma integration head-on. Ministers have made a unanimous commitment to improve the situation for Roma communities on the ground ... The key tools for Roma integration are now in Member States' hands and it is important that words are followed with action. We will not hesitate to remind EU countries of their commitments and make sure that they deliver.

Roma integration in European societies is an avowed goal, an ideal adopted by consensus. It is part of a kind of planned integration where European technocrats and national governments devise interventions and solutions for the strengthening of ties with mainstream culture. The avowed goal is narrowing the 'gap' between the dominant culture and Roma culture on key aspects of employment, housing, health and education. European documents on Roma integration portray the European Union as a collective of 'nations aspiring to justice ... with definite goals and aspirations in view' (Nussbaum, 2013, p. 117).

The only issue seems to be, as some authors argue (e.g. McGarry, 2012), that EU policy conflates redistribution and recognition goals for social justice, instead of recognizing it as a dilemma. EU policy places less emphasis on racism and the continuous discrimination of Roma. The European Union works with the principle of increased financial, legal and political accountability, and presents and treats the moral exclusion of Romanies in Europe as if it were a procedural problem. In doing so, it downplays moral exclusion as a key aspect of Roma's predicament in Europe.

The European Commission's preference for policies of 'harmony' and 'reducing the gap' (rather than anti-racism) presents various consequences. Whereas local, individual racism is recognized, any higher-order racisms are denied: racism that derives from national policy, institutional racism or systemic racism in society.[3]

Anti-discrimination and two models of social change

This does not mean that anti-discrimination measures are absent from European policy documents that outline actions needed to reduce the gap and ensure community harmony and cohesion. Anti-discrimination recommendations are very much part of the European thinking and planning for social justice, but they routinely present the 'solution' as a problem of reducing prejudices by raising awareness. A telling example is that of the EU legal framework for Roma integration (European Council, 2013) that recommends the implementation of measures to combat discrimination and prejudice against Roma that would include:

> raising awareness about the benefits of Roma integration both in Roma communities and among the general public; raising the general public's awareness of the diverse nature of societies, and sensitising public opinion to the inclusion problems Roma face, including, where relevant, by addressing those aspects in public education curricula and teaching materials; taking effective measures to combat anti-Roma rhetoric and hate speech, and addressing racist, stereotyping or otherwise stigmatising language or other behaviours that could constitute incitement to discrimination against Roma.
>
> (p. 9)

The EU legal framework also highlights the importance of collective action and emancipation, what the document calls 'empowerment':

> support the active citizenship of Roma by promoting their social, economic, political and cultural participation in society, including at the local level, since the active involvement and participation of Roma themselves, including through their representatives and organisations, is crucial for the improvement of their living conditions, as well as for the advancement of their social inclusion.
>
> (p. 10)

The two models of social change reflected in the EU legal framework document hint at a metatheory of integration in society where the cultivation of self-expression values of both majority and minority groups is paramount. Self-expression values are those values that promote tolerance and those that

Table 8.1 Two models of change (from Dixon *et al.*, 2012, p. 8)

Model of change	*Main agents of change*	*Interventions*	*Psychological processes*	*Behavioural outcome*
Prejudice-reduction model	Members of historically advantaged groups	Intergroup contact Cooperative interdependence Re-education Empathy arousal	Stereotype reduction More positive affect Decreased salience of group boundaries and identities	Reduction of individual acts of discrimination Reductions of intergroup conflict
Collective action model	Members of historically disadvantaged groups	Empowerment Consciousness raising Coalition building	Sense of injustice Collective anger Collective efficacy Increased salience of group boundaries and identities	Collective action to change the status quo

'motivate people to seek the civil and political rights that define liberal democracy' (Inglehart and Welzel, 2005, p. 152). It is assumed that social justice can be achieved by making people more open-minded and more aware of their biases, and by empowering minorities.

The general principles to which the EU legal document alludes reflect the two dominant models of social change in social psychology: the 'prejudice-reduction model' and the 'collective action model' of social change (Dixon *et al.*, 2012; Wright and Baray, 2012). The two models (see Table 8.1) are the most widely recognized means of tackling discrimination and inequalities and improving social relations, supported by a vast research literature.

Yet, as some social psychologists have shown, there are limits to both models of social change (cf. Dixon and Levine, 2012; Dixon *et al.*, 2012). The problem lies with the assumption that it is only a matter of method and approach to get 'people to like others more and to abandon their negative stereotypes' (Dixon *et al.*, 2012, p. 7). If negative evaluations are the problem, then 'raising awareness' (like in the case of the EU legal framework for Roma integration) is usually thought to be the solution. What takes priority is devising procedures for the 'emotional and cognitive rehabilitation of the advantaged' (Dixon and Levine, 2012, p. 315). Raising awareness can take many forms, but, for policy-makers, it is, essentially, an issue of more exposure, more education and internalization of positive images. Alongside raising awareness, collective mobilization of minority groups is seen as a much-needed ingredient.

The two models of change describe prejudice as a 'problem' that is the upshot of various combinations of psychological processes and fail to address directly societal aspects. The two models of change perpetuate a framework of addressing prejudice as an issue of intergroup relations (the main agents of change are either 'advantaged' or 'disadvantaged' groups), with the assumptions that groups operate, or are perceived, on a similar or an equal footing. Both models of change only partly engage with the societal complexity of prejudices, their history and symbolism, and implications for understanding social and societal mechanisms of moral exclusion that alter, transform or diminish the moral worth and dignity of people.

Particular prejudices, especially those whose consequence is harm inflicted by indignity, are not so easily amenable to psychological analysis. Although psychological analysis can indeed illuminate a range of very important aspects, it is limited in its understanding of prejudice as a social problem that manifests itself on many fronts. Social psychologists debate how to reconcile the two models of social change by arguing that

> efforts to change unjust and unequal social structures will require both harmony and managed conflict, a recognition of group differences as well as similarities, open discussion of existing inequalities that exposes both discrimination and privilege and enough animus and acrimony to stimulate assertive action.
>
> (Wright and Baray, 2012, p. 244)

Yet they do not discuss unjust and unequal relationships that are the outcome of how society, and its 'tests' of worth, relegate specific categories of people to a diminished, reduced moral status and worth. Pragmatic (policy) choices might not always imply a choice between harmony and conflict, might not always imply conventional intergroup dynamics between 'advantaged' and 'disadvantaged' groups. Some groups, like the Romanies, are perceived as a group apart from any other minority, 'disadvantaged' group.

As I argued in this book, Romanies are not only constantly degraded, but also constantly reminded of their degraded, inferior, transgressive, repulsive status. One cannot only understand this phenomenon by addressing prejudices not just as an issue of psychological processes but also as an issue that concerns more the dilemmas, contradictions, of mainstream liberal democratic society, and the actual clashes between (national and European) creed and actual practices.

Understanding the human and moral consequences of how European nation-states choose to meet the (national) challenges of solidarity and social cohesion must take into account some key characteristics of globalization. As Benhabib argues, 'globalization, insofar as it increases both the intensity and the interconnectedness of human actions around the world, results in the creation of new sites and new logics of representation' (2004, pp. 218–219). An emergent new site and logic of representation is the symbolism around *conditional* inclusion, solidarity and sympathy, especially in the hands of policy-makers and politicians.

The various pragmatic dimensions of planned social justice are the perfect ground for the perpetuation of conditional or ambiguous solidarity and sympathy. Politicians will preach equality of chances but will also remind everyone of pressures, constraints, etc., placed on imparting good will to others. The example below comes from the British Liberal Democrat politician Nick Clegg and former Labour Home Secretary, David Blunkett, adding their views to an ongoing conversation about potential inter-ethnic tensions between the local community and Roma migrants in the English city of Sheffield:

> We have every right to say if you are in Britain and are coming to live here and you are bringing up a family here, you have got to be sensitive to the way life is lived in this country. If you do things that people find intimidating, such as large groups hanging around on street corners, you have got to listen to what other people in the community say …
>
> I am a liberal. I think one of the great things about our country is that we are open-hearted and generous-minded. The NHS would keel over if it did not have people coming to this country to work for it. Of course we should welcome people that want to play by the rules, pay their taxes and contribute to public life.
>
> (Nick Clegg)

> We've got to be tough and robust in saying to people you are not in a downtrodden village or woodland, because many of them don't even live in areas where there are toilets or refuse collection facilities … You are not there any more, you are here – and you've got to adhere to our standards, and to our way of behaving, and if you do then you'll get a welcome and people will support you.
>
> (David Blunkett)

The two British politicians express a widely held belief – that firmness (resolve) and generosity (sympathy) are compatible. These two examples are very similar to the ones analysed in Chapter 6 – voices of reasonableness and rationality that present the Romanies as morally transgressive, 'out of place' and transgressors of fundamental moral values. The image of respectability and civility projected by these two accounts is at odds with the moral exclusionary implications of these accounts – that people like the Romanies are to be kept out at all costs, that rejection, discrimination and imposing limits on freedom of movement are reasonable, and necessary, reactions. Faced with different ways of being in the world and, more generally, with poverty and destitution, politicians across the political spectrum will erect boundaries and will ensure that the decency and rights of 'citizens' come first. The complaint that Clegg and Blunkett are airing is that Romanies do not seem to share the basic self-expression motivational drives that characterize advanced democratic societies (Inglehart and Welzel, 2005).

But what politicians like Clegg and Blunkett ignore is that those to whom firmness of law and generosity apply are what Roma historian, Sarah Carmona, calls 'a people multiple in themselves' but not in solidarity with mainstream society and the projects of the legislators and policy-makers. Clegg and Blunkett express the commonly shared European vision of Roma, the extreme ambivalence towards the Roma. Carmona, cited by *The New Yorker*, describes the European vision of Roma as 'paranoid and schizophrenic': 'They love our Gypsyness, our folklore, but hate our Romaniness. They claim to value our distinctiveness, and, at the same time, they cannot bear our abnormality' (Gopnik, 2014).

Stubborn prejudices and extending the social psychology of moral exclusion

A critical project in the social psychology of racism is already well under way (cf. Dixon and Levine, 2012). Social psychology has perhaps the most venerable and the most successful tradition of scientific analysis of social issues, yet systematic and reflexive analyses of the societal contradictions and dilemmas that contribute to the perpetuation of what Allport called 'stubborn' prejudices seem to elude social psychologists.

In this book I argued that taking full advantage of interdisciplinary affinities might open up social psychology to understanding racism as a social and cultural creation. The investigation of Roma issues continues to be a marginal concern in social psychology. It shows perhaps social psychology's reluctance to research programmatically historical and ideological prejudices. The study of 'stubborn' prejudices is left to the sociologist or political scientist. As I have shown in this book, the social psychologist who sets out to understand the nature and complexity of contemporary racism in Europe can profitably turn to sociology, social theory, anthropology and history to understand more about the dilemmas and contradictions lodged at the heart of liberal democratic societies.

This orientation presents several advantages. It allows social psychology (of racism) to include into its analyses those societal aspects that are crucial for understanding some of the major issues that permit the perpetuation of contemporary racism in Europe – national and globalized democratic governance, mechanisms for the extension of basic human rights to others, and mechanisms for the transformation, diminution or refusal of dignity. Furthermore, it can contribute to replacing an outdated conception of 'society' from social psychological theorizing, which bears little relation to how racism is actually perpetuated and enacted in society. The intellectual preoccupations of social psychologists of prejudice and racism reflect only partially societal issues, everyday, historical, political, legal, material aspects.

If prejudice is indeed an interpretive issue, then researching its psychological parameters is arguably not enough. In order to understand and judge the nature, diversity and intensity of prejudices one needs to perform not only psychological, but also cultural analysis; a cultural analysis of a society's presuppositions and its societal mechanisms of assigning, transforming or altering people's worth and dignity.

There is no racism or moral exclusion *outside of* culture. We need to take seriously the idea that one of the major sources of moral exclusion is a society's own moral evaluative schemes for judging people's dignity. Society can alter, transform, our own ideas about other people's human rights, our assessment of their safety and vulnerability, and our judgement about our own, and society's, role in oppression. Those who are perceived and construed as 'undeserving' are placed outside the bounds of solidarity and sympathy. That is why prejudice needs to be studied more as a societal and less as a psychological phenomenon. We must neither under- nor over-privilege cultural analysis in our analytical approaches. We must, however, ensure that we assign it to its rightful place.

In order to ensure that our theories are kept 'appropriately complex and attuned to real-world conditions' (Paluck and Green, 2009, p. 360), we need to bring to the understanding of racism a broader and more comprehensive understanding of the function of cultural analysis of how individuals, groups, communities transform the worth of others.

In this book I argued that the problems of prejudice and hostility in society are irreducible to flawed reasoning, irrational propensities and/or attitudinal negativity. Contemporary racism against Romanies in Europe wavers between the politics (and consequences) of extreme violence and the politics and consequences of a liberal humanist mentality that presents Romanies as transgressive and repulsive. In reality, most manifestations of racism pursue a middle course; racism is, more often than not, lukewarm, apathetic and ambivalent. And, more often than not, the liberal goal of 'eliminating' racism is no more than a 'diffuse' goal in 'the spirit of constitutional principles' (Nussbaum, 2013, p. 117). In our analyses of prejudice, we need to concern ourselves more with exploring the paradoxes lodged at the heart of the social expression of prejudice in liberal democracies. We must endeavour to interpret society as cultural and historical reality, which generates its own social processes and mechanisms of assigning moral significance to others.

Notes

1 I argued in Chapter 1 that the 'pervasiveness' and 'complexity' of explaining prejudice are not sufficient *appui* for understanding its particularities, distinctiveness and uniqueness in certain societies and conditions, and plural manifestations. The

majority of contemporary European puzzles that racism raises manifest themselves without the presence of deliberate hatred.

2 As Moscovici argues, the taboo of contact, 'an ancient and probably universal taboo … is always an obstacle to everyday encounters, and it objectifies behaviours of rejection, disgust or fear towards the minority' (2011, p. 455).

3 Roma activists and advocates, such as ERRC Executive Director Robert Kushen, highlighted the inadequacies of this intervention in a joint statement with the ERPC: 'Although we welcome the European Commission's direction to tackle Roma exclusion by defining concrete targets and timelines to address persistent and illegal school segregation, rampant unemployment, substandard housing and discrimination in access to health care, the Commission was silent on one critical impediment to Roma inclusion: anti-Gypsyism, which manifests itself in intimidation, harassment and violence against Roma. Unless States take forceful action against anti-Gypsyism, Roma will continue to be second-class citizens in Europe' (ERRC/ERPC, 2011).

Appendix

Transcription notations

(.)	Micro-pause
(2.0)	Pause length in seconds
[overlap]	Overlapping speech
°I know°	'Degree' signs enclose quieter speech
yes	Underlining indicates stress or emphasis in the speech
>faster<	Encloses speeded up talk
<slower>	Encloses speech delivered at slower pace
(clears throat)	Comments from the transcriber
=	'Equals' signs mark immediate 'latching' of successive talk
(…)	Shows where some talk has been omitted from a data extract
I do::n't	Colons mark degrees of elongation of the prior sound
Yeh,	Commas mark weak rising intonation
Yeh.	Stops mark stopping intonation

For a full list of transcription conventions, see Jefferson (2004).

References

About, I. (2012) 'Underclass Gypsies: An historical approach on categorization and exclusion in France in the nineteenth and twentieth centuries', in M. Stewart (ed.) *The Gypsy 'Menace': Populism and the New Anti-Gypsy Politics* (pp. 95–114), London: Hurst & Company.

Ackerman, N. W. and Jahoda, M. (1950) *Anti-Semitism and Emotional Disorder: A Psychoanalytic Interpretation*, New York: Harper and Brothers.

Adorno, T. W., Frenkel-Brunswik, E., Levinson, D. J. and Sanford, R. N. (1982 [1950]) *The Authoritarian Personality*, New York: Harper.

Allport, G. W. (1950) 'Prejudice: A problem in psychological and social causation', *Journal of Social Issues*, 6: 4–23.

Allport, G. W. (1954) *The Nature of Prejudice*, Reading, MA: Addison-Wesley.

Allport, G. W. (1960) *Personality and Social Encounter: Selected Essays*, Boston: Beacon Press.

Altemeyer, B. (1981) *Right-Wing Authoritarianism*, Winnipeg: University of Manitoba Press.

Amnesty International (2013) *Europe: Facts of Shame – Discrimination, Forced Evictions, Segregation and Violence against Roma in the European Union*, Public statement, April.

Amnesty International (2014) *'We Ask for Justice': Europe's Failure to Protect Roma from Racist Violence*, Amnesty International Report, April.

Anderson, K. (2009) *Benign Bigotry: The Psychology of Subtle Prejudice*, New York: Cambridge University Press.

Antaki, C. and Wetherell, M. (1999) 'Show concessions', *Discourse Studies*, 1: 7–27.

Appiah, K. A. (1994) 'Authenticity, survival: Multicultural societies and social reproduction', in A. Gutmann (ed.) *Multiculturalism: Examining the Politics of Recognition* (pp. 149–163), Princeton, NJ: Princeton University Press.

Arkes, H. R. and Tetlock, P. E. (2004) 'Attributions of implicit prejudice, or "Would Jesse Jackson 'fail' the Implicit Association Test?"', *Psychological Inquiry*, 15: 257–278.

Ashmore, R. and Del Boca, F. (1979) 'Sex stereotypes and implicit personality theory: Toward a cognitive-social psychological conceptualization', *Sex Roles*, 5: 219–248.

Asséo, H. (1994) *Les Tsiganes: Une Destinée Européenne*, Paris: Gallimard.

Augoustinos, M. (1998) 'Social representations and ideology: Towards the study of ideological representations', in U. Flick (ed.) *The Psychology of the Social* (pp. 156–169), Cambridge: Cambridge University Press.

Augoustinos, M. and Every, D. (2007) 'The language of "race" and prejudice: A discourse of denial, reason, and liberal-practical politics', *Journal of Language and Social Psychology*, 26: 123–141.

Augoustinos, M. and Every, D. (2010) 'Accusations and denials of racism: Managing moral accountability in public discourse', *Discourse & Society*, 21: 251–256.

Augoustinos, M. and Tileagă, C. (2012) 'Twenty five years of discursive psychology', *British Journal of Social Psychology*, 51: 405–412.

Augoustinos, M. and Walker, I. (1998) 'The construction of stereotypes within social psychology: From social cognition to ideology', *Theory & Psychology*, 8: 629–652.

Augoustinos, M., Tuffin, K. and Rapley, M. (1999) 'Genocide or failure to gel? Racism, history and nationalism in Australian talk', *Discourse and Society*, 10: 351–378.

Bain, P., Vaes, J. and Leyens, J. P. (2013) *Humanness and Dehumanization*, New York: Psychology Press.

Baker, D. (2012) *Bohemia Revisited*. Available online at www.theeuropean-magazine.com/daniel-baker–2/532-roma-in-europe (accessed March 2014).

Banaji, M. and Greenwald, A. (2013) *Blindspot: Hidden Biases of Good People*, New York: Delacorte Press.

Bandura, A. (1999) 'Moral disengagement in the perpetration of inhumanities', *Personality and Social Psychology Review*, 3: 193–209.

Barany, Z. (1998) 'Orphans of transition: Gypsies in eastern Europe', *Journal of Democracy*, 9: 142–156.

Barany, Z. (2002) *The East European Gypsies: Regime Change, Marginality and Ethnopolitics*, Cambridge: Cambridge University Press.

Barroso, J. M. (2014) 'Reforming Europe in a changing world', LSE European Institute and Department of Law public lecture, 14 February.

Bar-Tal, D. (1989) 'Delegitimization: The extreme case of stereotyping and prejudice', in D. Bar-Tal, C. Graumannn, A. W. Kruglanski and W. Stroebe (eds) *Stereotyping and Prejudice*, New York: Springer Verlag.

Bar-Tal, D. (1990) 'Causes and consequences of delegitimization: Models of conflict and ethnocentrism', *Journal of Social Issues*, 46: 65–81.

Bar-Tal, D. (2000) *Shared Beliefs in a Society: Social Psychological Analysis*, London: Sage.

Bar-Tal, D. and Teichman, Y. (2005) *Stereotypes and Prejudice in Conflict: Representations of Arabs in Israeli Jewish Society*, New York: Cambridge University Press.

Bastian, B. and Haslam, N. (2011) 'Experiencing dehumanization: Cognitive and emotional effects of everyday dehumanization', *Basic and Applied Social Psychology*, 33: 295–303.

Bastian, B., Laham, S., Wilson, S., Haslam, N. and Koval, P. (2011) 'Blaming, praising, and protecting our humanity: The implications of everyday dehumanization for judgments of moral status', *British Journal of Social Psychology*, 50: 469–483.

Bauman, Z. (1989) *Modernity and the Holocaust*, Ithaca, NY: Cornell University Press.

Bauman, Z. (1990) 'Effacing the face: On the social management of moral proximity', *Theory, Culture and Society*, 7: 5–38.

Bauman, Z. (1995) *Life in Fragments: Essays in Postmodern Morality*, Oxford and Cambridge, MA: Blackwell.

Beck, U. (2006) *Cosmopolitan Vision*, Cambridge: Polity Press.

Becker, H. (1963) *Outsiders: Studies in the Sociology of Deviance*, New York: The Free Press.

Becker, H. (1967) 'Whose side are we on?', *Social Problems*, 14: 239–247.

Benedik, S. (2010) 'Harming "cultural feelings": Images and categorization of temporary Romani migrants to Graz/Austria', in M. Stewart and M. Rövid (eds) *Multi-disciplinary Approaches to Romany Studies* (pp. 71–90), Budapest: Central European University Press.

Benhabib, S. (2004) *The Rights of Others: Aliens, Residents and Citizens*, Cambridge: Cambridge University Press.

Bergmann, J. R. (1998) 'Introduction: Morality in discourse', *Research on Language and Social Interaction*, 31: 279–294.

Berry, J. (2006) 'Contexts of acculturation', in D. Sam and J. Berry (eds) *The Cambridge Handbook of Acculturation Psychology* (pp. 27–42), New York: Cambridge University Press.

Bhabha, H. (1992) 'Postmodern authority and postmodern guilt', in L. Grossberg, C. Nelson and P. Treichler (eds) *Cultural Studies* (pp. 55–66), London: Routledge.

Billig, M. (1976) *Social Psychology and Intergroup Relations*, London: Academic Press.

Billig, M. (1978) *Fascists: A Social Psychological View of the National Front*, London: Academic Press.

Billig, M. (1985) 'Prejudice, categorisation and particularisation: From a perceptual to a rhetorical approach', *European Journal of Social Psychology*, 15: 79–103.

Billig, M. (1987) 'Anti-Semitic themes and the British Far Left: Some socio-psychological observations on indirect aspects of the conspiracy tradition', in C. F. Graumann and S. Moscovici (eds) *Changing Conceptions of Conspiracy*, New York: Springer Verlag.

Billig, M. (1988) 'The notion of "prejudice": Some rhetorical and ideological aspects', *Text*, 8: 91–111.

Billig, M. (1991) *Ideology and Opinions*, London: Sage.

Billig, M. (1992) *Talking of the Royal Family*, London: Routledge.

Billig, M. (1994) 'Re-populating the depopulated pages of social psychology', *Theory & Psychology*, 4: 307–335.

Billig, M. (1995) *Banal Nationalism*, London: Sage.

Billig, M. (1996) *Arguing and Thinking: A Rhetorical Approach to Social Psychology* (2nd edn), Cambridge: Cambridge University Press.

Billig, M. (1997) 'The dialogic unconscious: Psycho-analysis, discursive psychology and the nature of repression', *British Journal of Social Psychology*, 36: 139–159.

Billig, M. (1998) 'Rhetoric and the unconscious', *Argumentation*, 12: 199–216.

Billig, M. (1999) *Freudian Repression*, Cambridge: Cambridge University Press.

Billig, M. (2001) 'Humour and hatred: The racist jokes of the Ku Klux Klan', *Discourse & Society*, 12: 267–289.

Billig, M. (2002a) 'Henri Tajfel's "Cognitive aspects of prejudice" and the psychology of bigotry', *British Journal of Social Psychology*, 41: 171–188.

Billig, M. (2002b) 'A response to Brown and Frosh', *British Journal of Social Psychology*, 41: 199–202.

Billig, M. and Tajfel, H. (1973) 'Social categorization and similarity in intergroup behaviour', *European Journal of Social Psychology*, 3: 27–52.

Billig, M., Condor, S., Edwards, D., Gane, M., Middleton, D. and Radley, A. (1988) *Ideological Dilemmas: A Social Psychology of Everyday Thinking*, London: Sage.

Blackwood, L., Hopkins, N. and Reicher, S. (2013) 'I know who I am, but who do they think I am? Muslim perspectives on encounters with airport authorities', *Ethnic and Racial Studies*, 36: 1090–1108.

Blumer, H. (1998 [1969]) *Symbolic Interactionism: Perspective and Method*, Berkeley: University of California Press.

Blumer, H. (1971) 'Social problems as collective behavior', *Social Problems*, 18: 298–306.

Bobo, L., Kluegel, J. and Smith, R. (1997) 'Laissez-faire racism: The crystallization of a kinder, gentler, anti-black ideology', in S. Tuch and J. Martin (eds) *Racial Attitudes in the 1990s: Continuity and Change* (pp. 15–44), Praeger.

Bogardus, E. (1928) *Immigration and Race Attitudes*, Boston: DC Heath.

Boltanski, L. (2011) *On Critique: A Sociology of Emancipation*, Cambridge: Polity Press.

Boltanski, L. (2012) *Love and Justice as Competences*, Cambridge: Polity Press.

Boltanski, L. and Thévenot, L. (2006 [1991]) *On Justification: Economies of Worth* (trans. Catherine Porter), Princeton, NJ: Princeton University Press.

Bonilla-Silva, E. (2014) *Racism without Racists: Color-blind Racism and the Persistence of Racial Inequality in America* (4th edn), Lanham, MD: Rowman & Littlefield.

Bourhis, R. Y. and Giles, H. (1977) 'The language of intergroup distinctiveness', in H. Giles (ed.) *Language, Ethnicity and Intergroup Relations*, London: Academic Press.

Breakwell, G. (1978) 'Some effects of marginal social identity', in H. Tajfel (ed.) *Differentiation between Social Groups*, London: Academic Press.

Brewer, M. B. and Campbell, D. T. (1976) *Ethnocentrism and Intergroup Attitudes: East African Evidence*, New York: Sage.

Brown, R. (1965) *Social Psychology*, London: Collier-MacMillan.

Brown, R. (1995) *Prejudice: Its Social Psychology*, Oxford: Blackwell.

Brown, R. (2010) *Prejudice: Its Social Psychology* (2nd edn), Oxford: Wiley-Blackwell.

Brown, R. and Abrams, D. (1986) 'The effects of intergroup similarity and goal interdependence on intergroup attitudes and task performance', *Journal of Experimental Social Psychology*, 22: 78–92.

Buttny, R. (1997) 'Reported speech in talking race on campus', *Human Communication Research*, 23: 477–506.

Campbell, D. T. (1958) 'Common fate, similarity, and other indices of the status of aggregates of persons as social entities', *Behavioural Science*, 3: 14–25.

Cantle, T. (2008) *Community Cohesion: A New Framework for Race and Diversity* (2nd edn), London: Palgrave.

Cantor, N. and Mischel, W. (1979) 'Prototypes in person perception', *Advances in Experimental Social Psychology*, 12: 3–51.

Caprara, G. V., Schwartz, S., Capanna, C., Vecchione, M. and Barbaranelli, C. (2006) 'Personality and politics: Values, traits, and political choice', *Political Psychology*, 27: 1–28.

Carrithers, M. (2005) 'Anthropology as a moral science of possibilities', *Current Anthropology*, 46: 433–456.

Chalmers, A. (1999) *What Is This Thing Called Science?* (3rd edn), Maidenhead: Open University.

Chouliaraki, L. and Fairclough, N. (1999) *Discourse in Late Modernity: Rethinking Critical Discourse Analysis*, Edinburgh: Edinburgh University Press.

Christie, R. and Jahoda, M. (eds) (1954) *Studies in the Scope and Method of 'The Authoritarian Personality'*, New York: Free Press.

Cochrane, R. and Billig, M. (1984) '"I'm not National Front but..."', *New Society*, 68: 255–258.

Condor, S. (1988) '"Race stereotypes" and racist discourse', *Text*, 8: 69–91.

Condor, S. (1990) 'Social stereotypes and social identity', in D. Abrams and M. Hogg (eds) *Social Identity Theory: Constructive and Critical Advances* (pp. 230–249), Hemel Hempstead: Harvester Wheatsheaf.

Condor, S. (2006) 'Public prejudice as collaborative accomplishment: Towards a dialogic social psychology of racism', *Journal of Community and Applied Social Psychology*, 16: 1–18.

Condor, S. and Figgou, L. (2012) 'Rethinking the prejudice problematic: A collaborative cognition approach', in J. Dixon and M. Levine (eds) *Beyond Prejudice: Extending the Social Psychology of Conflict, Inequality and Social Change* (pp. 200–222), Cambridge: Cambridge University Press.

Condor, S., Abell, J., Figgou, L., Gibson, S. and Stevenson, C. (2006) '"They're not racist …": Prejudice denial, mitigation and suppression in dialogue', *British Journal of Social Psychology*, 45, 441–462.

Costi, N. (2010) 'The spectre that haunts Italy: The systematic criminalization of the Roma and the fears of the Heartland', *Romani Studies*, 20: 105–136.

Craig, K. (2002) 'Examining hate-motivated aggression: A review of the social psychological literature on hate crimes as a distinct form of aggression', *Aggression and Violent Behavior*, 7: 85–101.

Crandall, C., Eshelman, A. and O'Brien, L. (2002) 'Social norms and the expression and suppression of prejudice: The struggle for internalization', *Journal of Personality and Social Psychology*, 82: 359–378.

Crandall, C., Ferguson, M. and Bahns, A. (2013) 'When we see prejudice: The normative window and social change', in C. Stangor and C. Crandall (eds) *Stereotyping and Prejudice* (pp. 53–70), New York: Psychology Press.

Crowe, D. (2008) 'The Roma in post-communist Europe: Questions of ethnic conflict and ethnic peace', *Nationalities Papers*, 36: 521–552.

Csepeli, G. and Simon, D. (2004) 'Construction of Roma identity in Eastern and Central Europe: Perception and self-identification', *Journal of Ethnic and Migration Studies*, 30: 129–150.

Cuddy, A., Fiske, S. and Glick, P. (2007) 'The BIAS Map: Behaviors from intergroup affect and stereotypes', *Journal of Personality and Social Psychology*, 92: 631–648.

Cuddy, A., Fiske, S. and Glick, P. (2008) 'Warmth and competence as universal dimensions of social perception: The stereotype content model and the BIAS map', *Advances in Experimental Social Psychology*, 40: 61–149.

Cuddy, A., Fiske, S., Kwan, V., Glick, P., Demoulin, S., Leyens, J. P., *et al.* (2009) 'Stereotype content model across cultures: Towards universal similarities and some differences', *British Journal of Social Psychology*, 48: 1–33.

Darley, J. and Gross, P. (1983) 'A hypothesis-confirming bias in labeling effects', *Journal of Personality and Social Psychology*, 44: 20–33.

Dasgupta, N. and Stout, J. (2012) 'Contemporary discrimination in the lab and field: benefits and obstacles of full-cycle social psychology', *Journal of Social Issues*, 68: 399–412.

De Cillia, R., Reisigl, M. and Wodak, R. (1999) 'The discursive construction of national identities', *Discourse & Society* 10: 149–173.

Delanty, G. (2009) *The Cosmopolitan Imagination: The Renewal of Critical Social Theory*, Cambridge: Cambridge University Press.

Delors, J. (2011) 'In search of Europe: An interview with Jacques Delors', *Eurozine*. Available online at www.eurozine.com/articles/2011-07-01-delors-en.html (accessed July 2013).

Derks, B., Scheepers, D. and Ellemers, N. (eds) (2013) *Neuroscience of Prejudice and Intergroup Relations*, Hove: Psychology Press.

Deschamps, J.-C. and Doise, W. (1978) 'Crossed category membership in intergroup relations', in H. Tajfel (ed.) *Differentiation in Social Groups: Studies in the Social Psychology of Intergroup Relations* (pp. 141–158), London: Academic Press.

Devine, P. (1989) 'Stereotypes and prejudice: Their automatic and controlled components', *Journal of Personality and Social Psychology*, 56: 5–18.

Devine, P. (1995) 'Prejudice and out-group perception', in A. Tesser (ed.) *Advanced Social Psychology* (pp. 467–513), New York: McGraw-Hill.

Diab, L. N. (1959) 'Authoritarianism and prejudice in near-Eastern students attending American universities', *Journal of Social Psychology*, 50: 175–187.

Dixon, J. A. (2001) 'Contact and boundaries: "Locating" the social psychology of intergroup relations', *Theory & Psychology*, 11: 587–608.

Dixon, J. A. and Durrheim, K. (2000) 'Displacing place identity: A discursive approach to locating self and other', *British Journal of Social Psychology*, 39: 27–44.

Dixon, J. and Levine, M. (2012) *Beyond Prejudice: Extending the Social Psychology of Conflict, Inequality and Social Change*, Cambridge: Cambridge University Press.

Dixon, J., Foster, D. and Reicher, S. (1997) 'Ideology, geography and racial exclusion: The squatter camp as "blot on the landscape" ', *Text*, 17: 317–348.

Dixon, J., Levine, M., Reicher, S. and Durrheim, K. (2012) 'Beyond prejudice: Are negative evaluations the problem and is getting us to like one another more the solution?', *Behavioral and Brain Sciences*, 35: 1–56.

Dixon, J., Durrheim, K., Kerr, P. and Thomae, M. (2013) ' "What's so funny 'bout peace, love and understanding?" Further reflections on the limits of prejudice reduction as a model of social change', *Journal of Social and Political Psychology*, 1: 239–252.

Dovidio, J. and Fazio, R. H. (1992) 'New technologies for the direct and indirect assessment of attitudes', in J. M. Tanur (ed.) *Questions about Questions: Inquiries into the Cognitive Bases of Surveys*, New York: Russell Sage.

Dovidio, J. and Gaertner, S. (2004) 'Aversive racism', *Advances in Experimental Social Psychology*, 36: 1–51.

Dovidio, J., Kawakami, K. and Gaertner, S. (2002a) 'Implicit and explicit prejudice in interracial interaction', *Journal of Personality and Social Psychology*, 82: 62–68.

Dovidio, J., Gaertner, S., Kawakami, K. and Hodson, G. (2002b) 'Why can't we just get along? Interpersonal biases and interracial distrust', *Cultural Diversity and Ethnic Minority Psychology*, 8: 88–102.

Dovidio, J., Glick, P. and Rudman, L. (2005) *On the Nature of Prejudice: Fifty Years after Allport*, Malden, MA: Blackwell.

Drew, P. (1998) 'Complaints about transgression and misconduct', *Research on Language and Social Interaction*, 31: 295–325.

Drury, J. (2012) 'Prejudice is about politics: A collective action perspective', *Behavioral and Brain Sciences*, 35: 20–21.

Duckitt, J. (1991) 'The development and validation of a subtle racism scale in South Africa', *South African Journal of Psychology*, 21: 233–239.

Duckitt, J. (1992) 'Education and authoritarianism among English and Afrikaans-speaking white South Africans', *Journal of Social Psychology*, 132: 701–708.

Duckitt, J. (2013) 'Historical overview', in J. Dovidio, M. Hewstone, P. Glick and V. Esses (eds) *The SAGE Handbook of Prejudice, Stereotyping and Discrimination* (pp. 29–44), London: Sage.

Duckitt, J., Bizumic, B., Krauss, S. and Heled, E. (2010) 'A tripartite approach to right-wing authoritarianism: The authoritarianism-conservatism-traditionalism model', *Political Psychology*, 31: 685–715.

Duncan, B. (1976) 'Differential social perception and attribution of intergroup violence: Testing the lower limits of stereotyping Blacks', *Journal of Personality and Social Psychology*, 34: 590–598.

Durrheim, K. (2012) 'Implicit prejudice in mind and interaction', in J. Dixon and M. Levine (eds) *Beyond Prejudice: Extending the Social Psychology of Conflict, Inequality and Social Change* (pp. 179–199), Cambridge: Cambridge University Press.

Durrheim, K. (2014) 'Two histories of prejudice', in C. Tileagă and J. Byford (eds) *Psychology and History: Interdisciplinary Explorations* (pp. 205–222), Cambridge: Cambridge University Press.

Durrheim, K. and Dixon, J. (2000) 'Theories of culture in racist discourse', *Race and Society*, 3: 93–109.

Durst, J. (2010) '"What makes us Gypsies, who knows...?!": Ethnicity and reproduction', in M. Stewart and M. Rövid (eds) *Multi-disciplinary Approaches to Romany Studies* (pp. 13–34), Budapest: Central European University Press.

Dworkin, R. (2013) *Justice for Hedgehogs*, Cambridge, MA: Harvard University Press.

Eagleton, T. (1991) 'Discourse and ideology', in T. Eagleton, *Ideology: An Introduction* (pp. 193–220), London: Verso.

Edelman, M. (1977) *Political Language: Words That Succeed and Policies That Fail*, New York: Academic Press.

Edwards, D. (1991) 'Categories are for talking: On the cognitive and discursive bases of categorisation', *Theory & Psychology*, 1: 515–542.

Edwards, D. (1997) *Discourse and Cognition*, London: Sage.

Edwards, D. (2003) 'Analysing racial discourse: A view from discursive psychology', in H. van den Berg, H. Houtkoop Steenstra and M. Wetherell (eds) *Analyzing Interviews on Racial Issues: Multidisciplinary Approaches to Interview Discourse*, Cambridge: Cambridge University Press.

Edwards, D. and Potter, J. (1992) *Discursive Psychology*, London: Sage.

Erjavec, K. (2001) 'Media representation of the discrimination against the Roma in Eastern Europe: The case of Slovenia', *Discourse & Society*, 12: 699–727.

Essed, P. (1991) *Understanding Everyday Racism*, Newbury Park: Sage.

European Commission (2008) *Discrimination in the European Union: Perceptions, Experiences and Attitudes* (Special Barometer 296), July.

European Commission (2012) *Discrimination in the EU in 2012* (Special Eurobarometer 393), November.

European Council (2013) *Council Recommendation on Effective Roma Integration Measures in the Member States*, press release, December.

European Roma Rights Center [ERRC] (2014) *Census: Forced Evictions of Migrant Roma in France*, ERRC, January.

European Roma Rights Center/European Roma Policy Coalition (2011) *EU Framework Weak on Discrimination against Roma*, ERRC/ERPC, April.

Fairclough, N. (1989) *Language and Power*, London: Longman.

Fairclough, N. (1992) *Discourse and Social Change*, Cambridge: Polity Press.

Fairclough, N. (1995) *Critical Discourse Analysis*, London: Longman.

Fairclough, N. and Wodak, R. (1997) 'Critical discourse analysis', in T. A. van Dijk (ed.) *Discourse as Social Interaction: Discourse Studies – A Multidisciplinary Introduction* (vol. 2), London: Sage.

Fassin, D. (2005) 'Compassion and repression: The moral economy of immigration policies in France', *Cultural Anthropology*, 20: 362–387.

Fassin, D. (2006) 'Riots in France and silent anthropologists', *Anthropology Today*, 22: 1–3.

Fassin, D. (2008) 'Beyond good and evil? Questioning the anthropological discomfort with morals', *Anthropological Theory*, 8: 333–344.

Ferguson, N., Burgess, M. and Hollywood, I. (2008) 'Crossing the Rubicon: Deciding to become a paramilitary in Northern Ireland', *International Journal of Conflict and Violence*, 2: 130–137.

Figgou, L. and Condor, S. (2006) 'Irrational categorization, natural intolerance and reasonable discrimination: Lay representations of prejudice and racism', *British Journal of Social Psychology*, 45: 219–243.

Finkielkraut, A. (2013) *L'identité Malheureuse*, Paris: Stock.

Fiske, S. (2002) 'What we know about bias and intergroup conflict, the problem of the century', *Current Directions in Psychological Science*, 11: 123–128.

Fiske, S. and Molm, L. (2010) 'Bridging inequality from both sides now', *Social Psychology Quarterly*, 73: 341–346.

Fiske, S. and Taylor, S. (1991) *Social Cognition* (2nd edn), New York: McGraw Hill.

Fleck, G. and Rughinis, C. (eds) (2008) *Vino Mai Aproape: Incluziunea si Excluziunea Romilor in Societatea Romaneasca de Azi*, Agentia Nationala pentru Romi.

Fowler, R., Hodge, R., Kress, G. and Trew, T. (1979) *Language and Control*, London: Routledge & Kegan Paul.

Fraser, A. (1992) *The Gypsies*, Oxford: Blackwell.

Gaertner, S. L. and Dovidio, J. F. (1977) 'The subtlety of white racism, arousal and helping behaviour', *Journal of Personality and Social Psychology*, 35: 691–707.

Gaertner, S. L. and Dovidio, J. F. (1986) 'The aversive form of racism', in J. F. Dovidio and S. L. Gaertner (eds) *Prejudice, Discrimination and Racism* (pp. 61–90), Orlando, FL: Academic Press.

Gamson, W. A. (1992) *Talking Politics*, Cambridge: Cambridge University Press.

Glick, P. (2005) 'Choice of scapegoats', in J. Dovidio, P. Glick and L. Rudman (eds) *On the Nature of Prejudice: Fifty Years after Allport* (pp. 244–261), Malden, MA: Blackwell.

Glick, P. and Fiske, S. (2001) 'Ambivalent sexism', in M. P. Zanna (ed.) *Advances in Experimental Social Psychology* (vol. 33), Thousand Oaks, CA: Academic Press.

Goodman, S. and Burke, S. (2010) '"Oh you don't want asylum seekers, oh you're just racist": A discursive analysis of discussions about whether it's racist to oppose asylum seeking', *Discourse & Society*, 21: 325–340.

Goodman, S. and Rowe, L. (2014) '"Maybe it is prejudice... but it is NOT racism": Negotiating racism in discussion forums about Gypsies', *Discourse & Society*, 25: 132–146.

Gopnik, A. (2014) 'The people who pass: Pickpockets and paranoia in France', *The New Yorker*, 13 January. Available online at: www.newyorker.com/magazine/2014/01/13/the-people-who-pass.

Graumann, C. F. (1998) 'Verbal discrimination: A neglected chapter in the social psychology of aggression', *Journal for the Theory of Social Behaviour*, 28: 41–61.

Greenwald, A. G. and Banaji, M. R. (1995) 'Implicit social cognition: Attitudes, self-esteem, and stereotypes', *Psychological Review*, 102: 4–27.

Habermas, J. (2012) *The Crisis of the European Union: A Response*, Cambridge: Polity Press.

Hagendoorn L., Linssen H. and Tumanov, S. (2001) *Intergroup Relations in States of the Former Soviet Union: The Perception of Russians* (European Monographs in Social Psychology), Hove: Psychology Press.

Hamilton, D. and Trolier, T. (1986) 'Stereotypes and stereotyping: An overview of the cognitive approach', in J. F. Dovidio and S. L. Gaertner (eds) *Prejudice, Discrimination and Racism*, Orlando: Academic Press.

Hancock, I. (2002) *We Are the Romani People*, Hatfield: Centre de Recherches tsiganes/University of Hertfordshire Press.

Harré, R. and Secord, P. F. (1972) *The Explanation of Social Behaviour*, Oxford: Blackwell.

Harris, L. and Fiske, S. (2006) 'Dehumanizing the lowest of the low: Neuroimaging responses to extreme out-groups', *Psychological Science*, 17: 847–853.

Hasdeu, I. (2008) 'Imagining the Gypsy woman: Representations of Roma in Romanian museum', *Third Text*, 22: 347–357.

Haslam, N. and Loughnan, S. (2012) 'Prejudice and dehumanization', in J. Dixon and M. Levine (eds) *Beyond Prejudice: Extending the Social Psychology of Conflict, Inequality and Social Change* (pp. 89–104), Cambridge: Cambridge University Press.

Haslam, S. A. and Reynolds, K. (2012) 'All about us, but never about us: The three-pronged potency of prejudice', *Brain and Behavioral Sciences*, 35: 435–436.

Haslam, S. A. and Wilson, A. (2000) 'In what sense are prejudiced beliefs personal? The importance of ingroup shared stereotypes', *British Journal of Social Psychology*, 39: 45–63.

Henriques, J. (1984) 'Social psychology and the politics of racism', in J. Henriques, W. Hollway, C. Urwin, C. Venn and V. Walkerdine (eds) *Changing the Subject: Psychology, Social Regulation and Subjectivity* (pp. 60–89), London: Methuen.

Henwood, K. (1994) 'Resisting racism and sexism in academic psychology: A personal/political view', in K.- K. Bhavnani and A. Phoenix (eds) *Shifting Identities, Shifting Racisms* (pp. 41–62), London: Sage.

Henwood, K. and Phoenix, A. (1996) '"Race" in psychology: Teaching the subject', *Ethnic and Racial Studies*, 19: 841–863.

Hepburn, A. and Wiggins, S. (eds) (2007) *Discursive Research in Practice: New Approaches to Psychology and Interaction*, Cambridge: Cambridge University Press.

Hewstone, M., Rubin, M. and Willis, H. (2002) 'Intergroup bias', *Annual Review of Psychology*, 53: 575–604.

Hill, J. (2008) *The Everyday Language of White Racism*, Malden, MA: Wiley-Blackwell.

Hockenos, P. (1993) *Free to Hate: The Rise of the Right in Post-Communist Eastern Europe*, London: Routledge.

Hogg, M. A. and Abrams, D. (1988) *Social Identification: A Social Psychology of Intergroup Relations and Group Processes*, London: Routledge.

Honneth, A. (1996) *The Struggle for Recognition: The Moral Grammar of Social Conflicts*, Cambridge: Polity Press.

Hopkins, N. and Kahani-Hopkins, V. (2009) 'Reconceptualizing "extremism" and "moderation": From categories of analysis to categories of practice in the construction of collective identity', *British Journal of Social Psychology*, 48: 99–113.

Horvath, K. (2012) 'Silencing and naming the difference', in M. Stewart (ed.) *The Gypsy 'Menace': Populism and the New Anti-Gypsy Politics* (pp. 117–136), London: Hurst & Company.

Howarth, C. (2004) 'Re-presentation and resistance in the context of school exclusion: Reasons to be critical', *Journal of Community and Applied Social Psychology*, 14: 356–377.

IMAS (2009) *Barometrul Relatiilor Interetnice* (May–June 2009), Bucuresti.

Inglehart, R. and Welzel, C. (2005) *Modernization, Cultural Change, and Democracy: The Human Development Sequence*, Cambridge: Cambridge University Press.

Jackman, M. (1994) *The Velvet Glove: Paternalism and Conflict in Gender, Class and Race Relations*, Berkeley: University of California Press.

Jackman, M. (2001) 'License to kill: Violence and legitimacy in expropriative social relations', in J. Jost and B. Major (eds) *The Psychology of Legitimacy: Emerging Perspectives on Ideology, Justice, and Intergroup Relations* (pp. 437–468), New York: Cambridge University Press.

Jackman, M. (2005) 'Rejection or inclusion of outgroups?', in J. Dovidio, P. Glick and L. Rudman (eds) *On the Nature of Prejudice: Fifty Years after Allport* (pp. 89–105), Malden, MA: Blackwell.

Jahoda, G. (1999) *Images of Savages: Ancient Roots of Modern Prejudice in Western Culture*, New York: Routledge.

Jahoda, M. (1982) *Employment and Unemployment: A Social Psychological Analysis*, Cambridge: Cambridge University Press.

Jahoda, M., Lazarsfeld, P. and Zeisel, H. (1971) *Marienthal: A Sociography of an Unemployed Community*, Chicago: Aldine.

Jayyusi, L. (1991) 'Values and moral judgment: Communicative praxis as moral order', in G. Button (ed.) *Ethnomethodology and the Human Sciences* (pp. 227–251), Cambridge: Cambridge University Press.

Jayyusi, L. (1993) 'Premeditation and happenstance: The social construction of intention, action and knowledge', *Human Studies*, 16: 435–454.

Jefferson, G. (2004) 'Glossary of transcript symbols with an Introduction', in G. H. Lerner (ed.) *Conversation Analysis: Studies from the First Generation* (pp. 13–23), Philadelphia: John Benjamins.

Jones, J. M. (1997) *Prejudice and Racism* (2nd edn), New York: McGraw-Hill.

Jost, J. and Hamilton, D. (2005) 'Stereotypes in our culture', in J. Dovidio, P. Glick and L. Rudman (eds) *On the Nature of Prejudice: Fifty Years after Allport* (pp. 208–224), Malden, MA: Blackwell.

Jost, J., Banaji, M. and Nosek, B. (2004) 'A decade of system justification theory: Accumulated evidence of conscious and unconscious bolstering of the status quo', *Political Psychology*, 25: 881–919.

Jovchelovitch, S. (2007) *Knowledge in Context: Representations, Community and Culture*, London: Routledge.

Kabachnik, P. (2010a) 'England or Uruguay? The persistence of place and the myth of the placeless gypsy', *Area*, 42: 198–207.

Kabachnik, P. (2010b) 'Place invaders: Constructing the nomadic threat in England', *Geographical Review*, 100: 90–108.

Katz, D. and Braly, K. (1933) 'Racial stereotypes of one hundred college students', *Journal of Abnormal and Social Psychology*, 28: 280–290.
Katz, D. and Braly, K. (1935) 'Racial prejudice and racial stereotypes', *Journal of Abnormal and Social Psychology*, 30: 175–193.
Katz, I. and Hass, R. G. (1988) 'Racial ambivalence and American value conflict: Correlational and priming studies of dual cognitive structures', *Journal of Personality and Social Psychology*, 55: 893–905.
Katz, I., Wackenhut, J. and Hass, R. G. (1986) 'Racial ambivalence, value duality and behavior', in J. F. Dovidio and S. L. Gaertner (eds) *Prejudice, Discrimination and Racism* (pp. 35–59), Orlando, FL: Academic Press.
Kenrick, D. and Puxon, G. (2009) *Gypsies under the Swastika*, Hatfield: University of Hertfordshire Press.
Kinder, D. R. and Sanders, L. (1996) *Divided by Color*, Chicago: Chicago University Press.
Kinder, D. R. and Sears, D. O. (1981) 'Prejudice and politics: Symbolic racism versus racial threats to the good life', *Journal of Personality and Social Psychology*, 40: 414–431.
Klandermans, B. and Mayer, N. (2006) *Extreme Right Activists in Europe: Through the Magnifying Glass*, London: Routledge.
Kligman, G. (2001) 'On the social construction of "otherness": Identifying "the Roma" in post-socialist communities', *Review of Sociology*, 7: 61–78.
Kress, G. and Hodge, R. (1979) *Language as Ideology*, London: Routledge & Kegan Paul.
Kristeva, J. (1982) *Powers of Horror: An Essay on Abjection*, New York: Columbia University Press.
Kristeva, J. (1991) *Strangers to Ourselves*, New York: Columbia University Press.
Lane, R. (1962) *Political Ideology: Why the Common Man Believes What He Does*, New York: Free Press.
LeCouteur, A. and Augoustinos, M. (2001) 'The language of prejudice and racism', in M. Augoustinos and K. J. Reynolds (eds) *Understanding Prejudice, Racism and Social Conflict* (pp. 215–230), London: Sage.
Leudar, I. and Nekvapil, J. (2000) 'Presentations of Romanies in the Czech media: On category work in television debates', *Discourse & Society*, 11: 487–513.
Lewin, K. (1946) 'Action research and minority problems', *Journal of Social Issues*, 2: 34–46.
Leyens, J.-P. (2009) 'Retrospective and prospective thoughts about infrahumanization', *Group Processes & Intergroup Relations*, 12: 807–817.
Leyens, J.-P., Yzerbyt, V. and Schadron, G. (1994) *Stereotypes and Social Cognition*, London: Sage.
Leyens, J.-P., Paladino, P. M., Rodriguez-Torres, R., Vaes, J., Demoulin, S., Rodriguez-Perez, A. and Gaunt, R. (2000) 'The emotional side of prejudice: The attribution of secondary emotions to ingroups and outgroups', *Personality and Social Psychology Review*, 4: 186–197.
Leyens, J. -P., Cortes, B., Demoulin, S., Dovidio, J., Fiske, S., Gaunt, R., *et al.* (2003) 'Emotional prejudice, essentialism, and nationalism: The 2002 Tajfel Lecture', *European Journal of Social Psychology*, 33: 703–717.
Linell P. and Rommetveit, R. (1998) 'The many forms and facets of morality in dialogue: Epilogue for the Special Issue', *Research on Language and Social Interaction*, 31: 465–473.

Lippmann, W. (1922) *Public Opinion*, London: Allen & Unwin.

Ljujic, V., Vedder, P., Dekker, H. and van Geel, M. (2012) 'Romaphobia: A unique phenomenon?', *Romani Studies*, 22: 141–152.

Locke, V. and Johnston, L. (2001) 'Stereotyping and prejudice: A social cognitive approach', in M. Augoustinos and K. Reynolds (eds) *Understanding Prejudice, Racism and Social Conflict* (pp. 107–125), London: Sage.

Luke, M. A. and Maio, G. R. (2009) 'Oh the humanity! Humanity-esteem and its social importance', *Journal of Research in Personality*, 43: 586–601.

Lynn, N. and Lea, S. (2003) '"A phantom menace and the New Apartheid": The social construction of asylum-seekers in the United Kingdom', *Discourse & Society*, 14: 425–452.

McConahay, J. B. (1981) 'Reducing racial prejudice in desegregated schools', in W. D. Hawley (ed.) *Effective School Desegregation*, Beverley Hills, CA: Sage.

McConahay, J. B. (1982) 'Self-interest versus racial attitudes as correlates of anti-busing attitudes in Louisville: Is it the buses or the blacks?', *Journal of Politics*, 44: 692–720.

McConahay, J. B. (1986) 'Modern racism, ambivalence and the modern racism scale', in J. F. Dovidio and S. L. Gaertner (eds) *Prejudice, Discrimination and Racism*, Orlando, FL: Academic Press.

McConahay, J. B. and Hough, J. C. (1976) 'Symbolic racism', *Journal of Social Issues*, 32: 23–45.

McFarland, S. (2010a) 'Authoritarianism, social dominance, and other roots of generalized prejudice', *Political Psychology*, 31: 453–477.

McFarland, S. G. (2010b) 'Personality and support for universal human rights: A review and test of a structural model', *Journal of Personality*, 78: 1735–1763.

McFarland, S. (2011) 'The slow creation of humanity', *Political Psychology*, 32: 1–20.

McFarland, S. and Brown, D. (2008) 'Who believes that identification with all humanity is ethical?', *Psicologia Politica*, 36: 37–49.

McGarry, A. (2012) 'The dilemma of the European Union's Roma policy', *Critical Social Policy*, 32: 126–136.

MacLaughlin, J. (1998) 'Racism, ethnicity and multiculturalism in contemporary Europe: A review essay', *Political Geography*, 17: 1013–1024.

Marcu, A. and Chryssochoou, X. (2005) 'Exclusion of ethnic groups from the realm of humanity: Prejudice against the Gypsies in Britain and in Romania', *Psicologia Politica*, 30: 41–56.

Marcus, G. E. (ed.) (1998) *Critical Anthropology Now: Unexpected Contexts, Shifting Constituencies, Changing Agendas*, Santa Fe, NM: School of American Research Press.

Margalit, A. (1998) *The Decent Society*, Cambridge, MA: Harvard University Press.

Mărginean, I. (ed.) (2001) *Cercetări cu privire la Minoritatea Romă* [Research on the Roma], Bucuresti: Institutul de Cercetare a Calităţii Vièţii. Available online at www.rroma.ro.

Matras, Y. (2004) 'A conflict of paradigms: Review article of Barany, Zoltan, *The East-European Gypsies*; and Hancock, Ian, *We Are the Romani People*', *Romani Studies*, 14: 193–209.

Matras, Y. (2014) *I Met Lucky People: The Story of the Romani Gypsies*, London: Penguin.

Memmi, A. (1963) *Portrait of a Jew* (translated from the French by Elisabeth Abbott), London: Eyre & Spottiswoode.

Memmi, A. (2000) *Racism* (translated and with an Introduction by Steve Martinot; Foreword by Kwame Anthony Appiah), Minneapolis: University of Minnesota Press.

Merino, M. E. and Tileagă, C. (2011) 'The construction of ethnic minority identity: A discursive psychological approach to ethnic self-definition in action', *Discourse & Society*, 22: 86–101.

Minard, R. D. (1952) 'Race relations in the Pocahuntas coal field', *Journal of Social Issues*, 8: 29–44.

Misztal, B. (2012) 'The idea of dignity: Its modern significance', *European Journal of Social Theory*, 16: 101–121.

Mitchell, G. and Tetlock, P. E. (2006) 'Antidiscrimination law and the perils of mindreading', *Ohio State Law Journal*, 67: 1180–1192.

Mitten, R. and Wodak, R. (1993) 'On the discourse of racism and prejudice', *Folia Linguistica l*, 27(3–4): 192–215.

Mizsei, K. (2012) 'Robbing the Roma'. Available online at www.project-syndicate.org/commentary/the-growing-isolation-of-europe-s-roma-by-kalman-mizsei#sPBWUCCVCf6x3RqE.99 (accessed July 2013).

Moghaddam, F. M. (2012) 'The omnicultural imperative', *Culture & Psychology*, 18: 304–330.

Mondak, J. (2010) *Personality and the Foundations of Political Behavior*, New York: Cambridge University Press.

Moscovici, S. (1972) 'Theory and society in social psychology', in J. Israel and H. Tajfel (eds) *The Context of Social Psychology: A Critical Assessment* (pp. 17–68), London: Academic Press.

Moscovici, S. (1984) 'The phenomenon of social representations', in R. Farr and S. Moscovici (eds) *Social Representations* (pp. 3–70), Cambridge: Cambridge University Press.

Moscovici, S. (2011) 'An essay on social representations and ethnic minorities', *Social Science Information*, 50: 442–461.

Myrdal, G. (1996 [1944]) *An American Dilemma: The Negro Problem and Modern Democracy*, 2 vols, New Brunswick, NJ: Transaction Publishers.

Nacu, A. (2012) 'From silent marginality to spotlight scapegoating? A brief case study of France's policy towards the Roma', *Journal of Ethnic and Migration Studies*, 38: 1323–1328.

Newcomb, T. (1947) 'Autistic hostility and social reality', *Human Relations*, 1: 69–86.

Nicolae, V. (2009) *The Enemy Within: Roma, the Media and Hate Speech*. Available online at www.eurozine.com/articles/2009-03-20-nicolae-en.html (accessed July 2013).

Nicolae, V. (2012) *Roma Inclusion: Up to the Majority*. Available online at www.eurozine.com/articles/2012-02-24-nicolae-en.html (accessed July 2013).

Nier, J. and Gaertner, S. (2012) 'The challenge of detecting contemporary forms of discrimination', *Journal of Social Issues*, 68: 207–220.

Nordberg, C. (2006) 'Claiming citizenship: Marginalised voices on identity and belonging', *Citizenship Studies*, 10: 523–539.

Norman, K. (2004) 'Equality and exclusion: "Racism" in a Swedish town', *Ethnos*, 69: 204–228.

Nussbaum, M. (2013) *Political Emotions*, Cambridge, MA: Belknap Press.

Oakes, P. J. and Haslam, S. A. (2001) 'Distortion vs. meaning: Categorization on trial for inciting intergroup hatred', in M. Augoustinos and K. Reynolds (eds) *Understanding Prejudice, Racism and Social Conflict* (pp. 179–194), London: Sage.

Okely, J. (1983) *The Traveller-Gypsies*, Cambridge: Cambridge University Press.

Okely, J. (2010) 'Constructing culture through shared location, bricolage and exchange: The case of Gypsies and Roma', in M. Stewart and M. Rövid (eds) *Multi-disciplinary Approaches to Romany Studies* (pp. 71–90), Budapest: Central European University Press.

Olivera, M. (2012) 'Les Tsiganes comme autochtones: Le cas des Roms Gabori – Roumanie', *Balkanologie*, 14(1–2). Available online at http://balkanologie.revues.org/2340 (accessed August 2013).

Onraet, E. and van Hiel, A. (2014) 'Are right-wing adherents mentally troubled? Recent insights on the relationship of right-wing attitudes with threat and psychological ill-being', *Current Directions in Psychological Science*, 20: 35–40.

Open Society Institute (2011) *Beyond Rhetoric: Roma Integration Roadmap for 2020*, Budapest, June.

Opotow, S. (2007) 'Commentary: Moral exclusion and torture – The ticking bomb scenario and the slippery ethical slope', *Peace and Conflict: Journal of Peace Psychology*, 13: 457–461.

Opotow, S. (2011) 'How this was possible: Interpreting the Holocaust', *Journal of Social Issues*, 67: 205–224.

Paladino, P. M., Leyens, J. -P., Rodriguez, R., Rodriguez, A., Gaunt, R. and Demoulin, S. (2002) 'Differential association of uniquely and non-uniquely human emotions to the ingroup and the outgroups', *Group Processes and Intergroup Relations*, 5: 105–117.

Paluck, E. (2009) 'Reducing intergroup prejudice and conflict using the media: A field experiment in Rwanda', *Journal of Personality and Social Psychology*, 96: 574–587.

Paluck, E. L. and Green, D. P. (2009) 'Prejudice reduction: What do we know? A critical look at evidence from the field and the laboratory', *Annual Review of Psychology*, 60: 339–367.

Pedersen, A. and Walker, I. (1997) 'Prejudice against Australian Aborigines: Old fashioned and modern forms', *European Journal of Social Psychology*, 27: 561–587.

Perelman, C. and Olbrechts-Tyteca, L. (1971) *The New Rhetoric*, Notre Dame, IN: University of Notre Dame Press.

Pérez, J. A., Moscovici, S. and Chulvi, B. (2002) 'Natura y cultura como principio de clasificación social: Anclaje de representaciones sociales sobre minorías étnicas', *Revista de Psicología Social*, 17: 51–67.

Pettigrew, T. F. (1958) 'Personality and socio-cultural factors in inter-group attitudes: A cross-national comparison', *Journal of Conflict Resolution*, 2: 29–42.

Pettigrew, T. F. (1979) 'The ultimate attribution error: Extending Allport's cognitive analysis of prejudice', *Personality and Social Psychology Bulletin*, 5: 461–476.

Pettigrew, T. F. (1996) *How to Think Like a Social Scientist*, New York: HarperCollins.

Pettigrew, T. F. (2007) 'Still a long way to go: American Black–White relations today', in G. Adams, M. Biernat, N. Branscombe, C. Crandall and L. Wrightsman (eds) *Commemorating Brown: The Social Psychology of Racism and Discrimination* (pp. 45–61), Washington, DC: APA Press.

Pettigrew, T. F. and Meertens, R. W. (1995) 'Subtle and blatant prejudice in Western Europe', *European Journal of Social Psychology*, 25: 57–75.

Pettigrew, T. F., Jackson, J. S., Ben Brika, J., Lemaine, G., Meertens, R., Wagner, U. and Zick, A. (1998) 'Outgroup prejudice in Western Europe', *European Review of Social Psychology*, 8: 241–273.

Petrova, D. (2003) 'The Roma: Between a myth and the future', *Social Research*, 70: 111–161.

Pickering, M. (2001) *Stereotyping: The Politics of Representation*, New York: Palgrave.

Potter, J. (2012) 'Re-reading discourse and social psychology: Transforming social psychology', *British Journal of Social Psychology*, 51: 436–455.

Potter, J. and Hepburn, A. (2005) 'Qualitative interviews in psychology: Problems and possibilities', *Qualitative Research in Psychology*, 2: 1–27.

Potter, J. and Wetherell, M. (1987) *Discourse and Social Psychology: Beyond Attitudes and Behaviour*, London: Sage.

Potter, J. and Wetherell, M. (1988) 'Accomplishing attitudes: Fact and evaluation in racist discourse', *Text*, 8: 51–68.

Quasthoff, U. (1978) 'The uses of stereotype in everyday argument', *Journal of Pragmatics*, 2: 1–48.

Quasthoff, U. (1989) 'Social prejudice as a resource of power: Towards the functional ambivalence of stereotypes', in R. Wodak (ed.) *Language, Power and Ideology: Studies in Political Discourse*, Amsterdam: Benjamins.

Rapley, M. (2001) '"How to do X without doing Y": Accomplishing discrimination without "being racist" – "doing equity"', in M. Augoustinos and K. J. Reynolds (eds) *Understanding Prejudice, Racism and Social Conflict* (pp. 231–250), London: Sage.

Reeves, F. (1983) *British Racial Discourse*, Cambridge: Cambridge University Press.

Reicher, S. (2004) 'The context of social identity: Domination, resistance, and change', *Political Psychology*, 25: 921–945.

Reicher, S. (2011) 'Promoting a culture of innovation: BJSP and the emergence of new paradigms in social psychology', *British Journal of Social Psychology*, 50: 391–398.

Reicher, S. (2012) 'From perception to mobilization: The shifting paradigm of prejudice', in J. Dixon and M. Levine (eds) *Beyond Prejudice: Extending the Social Psychology of Conflict, Inequality and Social Change* (pp. 27–47), Cambridge: Cambridge University Press.

Reisigl, M. and Wodak, R. (2001) *Discourse and Discrimination: Rhetorics of Racism and Antisemitism*, London: Routledge.

Reynolds, K. J. and Turner, J. (2001) 'Prejudice as a group process: The role of social identity', in M. Augoustinos and K. Reynolds (eds) *Understanding Prejudice, Racism and Social Conflict* (pp. 159–178), London: Sage.

Reynolds, K. J. and Turner, J. C. (2006) 'Individuality and the prejudiced personality', *European Review of Social Psychology*, 17: 233–270.

Reynolds, K., Haslam, A. and Turner, J. (2012) 'Prejudice, social identity and social change: Resolving the Allportian problematic', in J. Dixon and M. Levine (eds) *Beyond Prejudice: Extending the Social Psychology of Conflict, Inequality and Social Change* (pp. 48–69), Cambridge: Cambridge University Press.

Ricoeur, P. (1986) *Lectures on Ideology and Utopia* (ed. by G. H. Taylor), New York: Columbia University Press.

Ridgeway, C. (2014) 'Why status matters for inequality', *American Sociological Review*, 79: 1–16.

Rokeach, M. (1956) 'Political and religious dogmatism: An alternate to the authoritarian personality', *Psychological Monographs*, 70(18): 1–43.
Rokeach, M. (1960) *The Open and Closed Mind*, New York: Basic Books.
Rorty, R. (1989) *Contingency, Irony and Solidarity*, Cambridge: Cambridge University Press.
Rosenthal, R. and Jacobson, L. (1968) *Pygmalion in the Classroom: Teacher Expectations and Student Intellectual Development*, New York: Holt, Rinehart and Winston.
Rosenwein, B. (2006) *Emotional Communities in the Early Middle Ages*, Ithaca, NY: Cornell University Press.
Rowe, L. and Goodman, S. (2014) '"A stinking filthy race of people inbred with criminality": A discourse analysis of prejudicial talk about Gypsies in discussion forums', *Romani Studies*, 24: 25–42.
Rudman, L. (2005) 'Rejection of women? Beyond prejudice as antipathy', in J. Dovidio, P. Glick and L. Rudman (eds) *On the Nature of Prejudice: Fifty Years after Allport* (pp. 106–120), Malden, MA: Blackwell
Rughiniş, C. (2012) *Masurarea sociologica: Teorii si practici ale cuantificarii*, Bucuresti: Polirom.
Sahlins, M. (2004) *Apologies to Thucydides: Understanding History as Culture and Vice Versa*, Chicago: University of Chicago Press.
Sampson, E. (1993) *Celebrating the 'Other': A Dialogic Account of Human Nature*, Boulder, CO: Westview.
Sartre, J. P. (1995 [1948]) *Anti-Semite and Jew: An Exploration of the Etiology of Hate*, New York: Schocken Books.
Schaller, M. and Neuberg, S. (2012) 'Danger, disease, and the nature of prejudice(s)', *Advances in Experimental Social Psychology*, 46: 1–54.
Schegloff, E. (2005) 'On complainability', *Social Problems*, 52: 449–476.
Sears, D. O. (1988) 'Symbolic racism', in P. A. Katz and D. A. Taylor (eds) *Eliminating Racism: Profiles in Controversy* (pp. 53–84), New York: Plenum Press.
Sears, D. O. and Kinder, D. R. (1971) 'Racial tensions and voting in Los Angeles', in W. Z. Hirsch (ed.) *Los Angeles: Viability and Prospects for Metropolitan Leadership* (pp. 51–88), New York: Praeger.
Sibley, D. (1992) 'Outsiders in society and space', in K. Anderson and F. Gale (eds) *Inventing Places: Studies in Cultural Geography* (pp. 107–122), Melbourne: Longman.
Sibley, D. (1994) 'The sin of transgression', *Area*, 26: 300–303.
Sibley, D. (1995) *Geographies of Exclusion: Society and Difference in the West*, London: Routledge.
Sibley, C. and Duckitt, J. (2008) 'Personality and prejudice: A meta-analysis and theoretical review', *Personality and Social Psychology Review*, 12: 248–279.
Sidanius, J. and Pratto, F. (1999) *Social Dominance: An Intergroup Theory of Social Hierarchy and Oppression*, New York: Cambridge University Press.
Siegel, A. E. and Siegel, S. (1957) 'Reference groups, membership groups and attitude change', *Journal of Abnormal and Social Psychology*, 55: 360–364.
Sigona, N. (2003) '"How can a nomad be a refugee?": Kosovo Roma and labelling policy in Italy', *Sociology*, 37: 69–79.
Sigona, N. and Trehan, N. (2009) 'Introduction: Romani politics in neoliberal Europe', in Sigona, N. and Trehan, N. (eds) *Romani Politics in Europe: Poverty, Ethnic Marginalisation and the Neoliberal Order* (pp. 1–22), Basingstoke: Palgrave.

Smith, D. (2006) *Globalization: The Hidden Agenda*, Cambridge: Polity Press.

Soros, G. (2013) *Empowering Europe's Roma*. Available online at www.project-syndicate.org/commentary/george-soros-argues-that-euope-s-roma-problem-is-increasingly-becoming-a-long-term-prosperity-problem#Pk9le5j0hIwvvkvD.99 (accessed July 2013).

Speer, S. and Potter, J. (2000) 'The management of heterosexist talk: Conversational resources and prejudiced claims', *Discourse & Society*, 11: 543–572.

Stenner, K. (2005) *The Authoritarian Dynamic*, Cambridge: Cambridge University Press.

Stephan, W. (1985) 'Intergroup relations', in G. Lindzey and E. Aronson (eds) *The Handbook of Social Psychology* (vol. 2), New York: Random House.

Stephan, W., Ybarra, O., Martinez, C., Schwarzwald, J. and Tur-Kaspa, M. (1998) 'Immigrants to Spain and Israel: An integrated threat theory analysis', *Journal of Cross-Cultural Psychology*, 29: 559–576.

Stephan, W. G., Diaz-Loving, R. and Duran, A. (2000) 'Integrated threat theory and intercultural attitudes: Mexico and the United States', *Journal of Cross-Cultural Psychology*, 31: 240–249.

Stephan, W. G., Boniecki, K. A., Ybarra, O., Bettencourt, A., Ervin, K. S., Jackson, L. A., McNatt, P. C. and Renfro, C. L. (2002) 'The role of threats in racial attitudes of Blacks and Whites', *Personality and Social Psychology Bulletin*, 28: 1242–1254.

Stephan, W. G., Renfro, C. L. and Davis, M. D. (2008) 'The role of threat in intergroup relations', in U. Wagner, L. R. Tropp, G. Finchilescu and C. Tredoux (eds) *Improving Intergroup Relations: Building on the Legacy of Thomas F. Pettigrew* (pp. 55–72), Oxford: Blackwell.

Stewart, M. (2012a) 'Foreword: New forms of anti-Gypsy politics – A challenge for Europe', M. Stewart (ed.) *The Gypsy 'Menace': Populism and the New Anti-Gypsy Politics*, London: Hurst & Co.

Stewart, M. (2012b) 'Populism, Roma and the European politics of cultural difference', in M. Stewart (ed.) *The Gypsy 'Menace': Populism and the New Anti-Gypsy Politics* (pp. 3–24), London: Hurst & Co.

Stokoe, E. (2009) 'Doing actions with identity categories: Complaints and denials in neighbour disputes', *Text & Talk*, 29: 75–97.

Stokoe, E. and Edwards, D. (2007) '"Black this, black that": Racial insults and reported speech in neighbor complaints and police interrogations', *Discourse & Society*, 18: 337–372.

Stroebe, W. and Insko, C. A. (1989) 'Stereotype, prejudice and discrimination: Changing conceptions in theory and research', in D. Bar-Tal, C. F. Graumann, A. W. Kruglanski and W. Stroebe (eds) *Stereotypes and Prejudice: Changing Conceptions* (pp. 3–34), Berlin: Springer.

Sykes, M. (1985) 'Discrimination in discourse', in T. A. van Dijk (ed.) *Handbook of Discourse Analysis* (vol. 4), London: Academic Press.

Tábori, Z. (2009) *Guns, Fire and Ditches: A Report from Tatárszentgyörgy on the Roma Killings*. Available online at www.eurozine.com/articles/2009-12-15-tabori-en.html (accessed July 2013).

Taguieff, P.-A. (1987) *La Force du Préjugé: Essai sur le Racisme et ses Doubles*, Paris: Gallimard.

Tajfel, H. (1978) *Differentiation Between Social Groups: Studies in the Social Psychology of Intergroup Relations*, London: Academic Press.

Tajfel, H. (1981a) 'Cognitive aspects of prejudice', in H. Tajfel, *Human Groups and Social Categories* (pp. 127–142), Cambridge: Cambridge University Press.
Tajfel, H. (1981b) 'Social stereotypes and social groups', in J. C. Turner and H. Giles (eds) *Intergroup Behaviour* (pp. 144–167), Oxford: Blackwell.
Tajfel, H. and Turner, J. (1986) 'The social identity theory of intergroup behaviour', in S. Worchel and W. G. Austin (eds) *Psychology of Intergroup Relations* (pp. 7–24), Chicago: Nelson Hall.
Tajfel, H. and Wilkes, A. L. (1963) 'Classification and quantitative judgment', *British Journal of Psychology*, 54: 101–114.
Tajfel, H., Flament, C., Billig, M. and Bundy, R. P. (1971) 'Social categorization and intergroup behaviour', *European Journal of Social Psychology*, 1: 149–178.
Taylor, C. (1994) 'The politics of recognition', in A. Gutmann (ed.) *Multiculturalism: Examining the Politics of Recognition* (pp. 25–74), Princeton, NJ: Princeton University Press.
Tetlock, P. E. and Mitchell, G. (2009) 'Implicit prejudice and accountability systems: What must organizations do to prevent discrimination?', *Research in Organizational Behavior*, 29: 3–38.
Thompson, J. B. (1984) *Studies in the Theory of Ideology*, Cambridge: Polity.
Thompson, J. B. (1987) 'Language and ideology: A framework for analysis', *Sociological Review*, 35: 516–536.
Thompson, J. B. (1990) *Ideology and Modern Culture*, Cambridge: Polity Press.
Tietze, N. and Bielefeld, U. (2010) 'In search of Europe: An interview with J. Delors'. Available online at www.pro-europa.eu/index.php/en/at-issue/the-way-to-the-future/28-in-search-of-europe-an-interview-with-j-delors.
Tileagă, C. (2005) 'Accounting for extreme prejudice and legitimating blame in talk about the Romanies', *Discourse & Society*, 16: 603–624.
Tileagă, C. (2006) 'Representing the "other": A discursive analysis of prejudice and moral exclusion in talk about Romanies', *Journal of Community and Applied Social Psychology*, 16: 19–41.
Tileagă, C. (2007) 'Ideologies of moral exclusion: A critical discursive reframing of depersonalization, delegitimization and dehumanization', *British Journal of Social Psychology*, 46: 717–737.
Tileagă, C. (2013) *Political Psychology: Critical Perspectives*, Cambridge: Cambridge University Press.
Tileagă, C. (2014) 'Prejudice as collective definition: Ideology, discourse and moral exclusion', in C. Antaki and S. Condor (eds) *Rhetoric, Ideology and Social Psychology: Essays in Honour of Michael Billig*, London: Routledge.
Tileagă, C. and Stokoe, E. (in press) *Discursive Psychology: Classic and Contemporary Issues*, London: Routledge.
Triandis, H. and Triandis, L. (1962) 'A cross-cultural study of social distance', *Psychological Monographs: General and Applied*, 76: 1–21.
Turner, J. (1999a) 'The prejudiced personality and social change: A self-categorization perspective', the Tajfel Lecture at the European Association of Experimental Social Psychology, Oxford, 7–11 July.
Turner, J. (1999b) 'Some current themes in research on social identity and self-categorization theories', in N. Ellemers, R. Spears and B. Doosje (eds) *Social Identity: Context, Commitment, Content* (pp. 6–34), Oxford: Blackwell.
Turner, J. and Reynolds, K. (2003) 'Why social dominance theory has been falsified', *British Journal of Social Psychology*, 42: 199–206.

Turner, J., Hogg, M. A., Oakes, P. J., Reicher, S. and Wetherell, M. (1987) *Rediscovering the Social Group: A Self-Categorization Theory*, Oxford and New York: Basil Blackwell.
van Dijk, T. A. (1984) *Prejudice and Discourse*, Amsterdam: Benjamins.
van Dijk, T. A. (1987) *Communicating Racism: Ethnic Prejudice in Thought and Talk*, London: Sage.
van Dijk, T. A. (1991) *Racism and the Press*, London: Routledge.
van Dijk, T. A. (1992) 'Discourse and the denial of racism', *Discourse & Society*, 3: 87–118.
van Dijk, T. A. (1993) *Elite Discourse and Racism*, Newbury Park, CA: Sage.
van Dijk, T. A. (1998) *Ideology: A Multidisciplinary Approach*, London: Sage.
van Dijk, T. A., Ting-Toomey, S., Smitherman, G. and Troutman, D. (1997) 'Discourse, ethnicity, culture and racism', in T. A. van Dijk (ed.) *Discourse as Social Interaction* (pp. 144–180), London: Sage.
van Leeuwen, T. and Wodak, R. (1999) 'Legitimising immigration control: A discourse- historical approach', *Discourse Studies*, 1: 83–118.
Verkuyten, M. (1997) 'Discourses of ethnic minority identity', *British Journal of Social Psychology*, 36: 565–586.
Verkuyten, M. (2001) '"Abnormalization" of ethnic minorities in conversation', *British Journal of Social Psychology*, 40: 257–278.
Verkuyten, M. (2003) 'Discourses about ethnic group (de-)essentialism: Oppressive and progressive aspects', *British Journal of Social Psychology*, 42: 371–391.
Verkuyten, M. and deWolf, A. (2002) 'Being, feeling and doing: Discourses and ethnic self-definitions among minority group members', *Culture & Psychology*, 8: 371–399.
Verkuyten, M. and Hagendoorn, L. (1998) 'Prejudice and self-categorisation: The variable role of authoritarianism and in-group stereotypes', *Personality and Social Psychology Bulletin*, 24: 99–110.
Verkuyten, M., De Jong, W. and Masson, C. N. (1995) 'The construction of ethnic categories: Discourses of ethnicity in the Netherlands', *Ethnic and Racial Studies*, 18: 251–276.
Verseck, K. (2013) 'Hungary's racism problem: Orbán friend says Roma "Shouldn't be allowed to exist"', *Spiegel Online*, 11 January. Available online at www.spiegel.de/international/europe/hungarian-journalist-says-roma-should-not-be-allowed-to-exist-a-876887.html.
Vincze, E. (2013) 'Socio-spatial marginality of Roma as form of intersectional justice', *Sociologia*, 2: 217–242.
Wacquant, L. (2008) *Urban Outcasts: A Comparative Sociology of Advanced Marginality*, Cambridge: Polity Press.
Wagner, U., Christ, O. and Heitmeyer, W. (2013) 'Anti-immigration bias', in J. Dovidio, M. Hewstone, P. Glick and V. Esses (eds) *The SAGE Handbook of Prejudice, Stereotyping and Discrimination* (pp. 361–377), London: Sage.
Wetherell, M. (1998) 'Positioning and interpretative repertoires: Conversation analysis and post-structuralism in dialogue', *Discourse & Society*, 9: 387–412.
Wetherell, M. (1999) 'Beyond binaries', *Theory & Psychology*, 9: 399–406.
Wetherell, M. (2001) 'Debates in discourse research', in M. Wetherell, S. Taylor and S. J. Yates (eds) *Discourse Theory and Practice: A Reader*, London: Sage and Open University.

Wetherell, M. (2012) *Affect and Emotion: A New Social Science Understanding*, London: Sage.

Wetherell, M. and Potter, J. (1992) *Mapping the Language of Racism: Discourse and the Legitimation of Exploitation*, Hemel Hempstead: Harvester Wheatsheaf.

Whitehead, K. (2009) '"Categorizing the categorizer": The management of racial common sense in interaction', *Social Psychology Quarterly*, 72: 325–342.

Widdicombe, S. and Wooffitt, R. (1995) *The Language of Youth Subcultures: Social Identity in Action*, Hemel Hempstead: Harvester/Wheatsheaf.

Wieviorka, M. (1995) *The Arena of Racism* (transl. Chris Turner), London: Sage.

Wieviorka, M. (1998) 'Is multiculturalism the solution?', *Ethnic and Racial Studies*, 21: 881–910.

Wiggins, S. and Potter, J. (2003) 'Attitudes and evaluative practices: Category vs. item and subjective vs. objective constructions in everyday food assessments', *British Journal of Social Psychology*, 42: 513–531.

Wodak, R. and Matouschek, B. (1993) '"We are dealing with people whose origins one can clearly tell just by looking": Critical discourse analysis and the study of neo-racism in contemporary Austria', *Discourse & Society*, 4: 225–248.

Wodak, R. and Reisigl, M. (1999) 'Discourse and racism: European perspectives', *Annual Review of Anthropology*, 28: 175–199.

Wodak, R., de Cillia, R., Reisgl, M. and Liebhart, K. (1999) *The Discursive Construction of National Identity*, Edinburgh: Edinburgh University Press.

Wright, S. and Baray, G. (2012) 'Models of social change in social psychology: Collective action or prejudice reduction? Conflict or harmony?', in J. Dixon and M. Levine (eds) *Beyond Prejudice: Extending the Social Psychology of Conflict, Inequality and Social Change* (pp. 225–247), Cambridge: Cambridge University Press.

Zachos, D. (2011) 'Sedentary Roma (Gypsies): The case of Serres (Greece)', *Romani Studies*, 21: 23–56.

Zerubavel, E. and Smith, E. (2010) 'Transcending cognitive individualism', *Social Psychology Quarterly*, 73: 321–325.

Index

Page numbers with 't' are tables.